Praise for JUST a LUMP IN THE ROAD ...

"Theirs is a woman-meets-woman, woman battles breast cancer type of tale. The book aims to help all the women now battling breast cancer."
—*The Palm Beach Post*

"They shared emotions and the physical side affects of drugs. They took care of each other in ways doctors did not."
—*The Ft. Lauderdale Sun-Sentinel*

"The real deal on what happens when your life and dreams are stopped in their tracks and how friendship can beat back cancer. This is a wonderful book written with care for others, as they search inside themselves for the courage and the spirit to go on day to day. This book helps those of us watching from the outside wondering just HOW DO WE HELP? WHAT CAN WE DO FOR OUR FRIENDS? ... read this and know."
—Steve Harmon, "The Breakfast Club"
KODJ Radio, Salt Lake City

"... a compelling compilation of six stories written by courageous young survivors from South Florida who have "been there".
—"Komen South Florida Affiliate"
eNewsletter, March 2008

JUST a LUMP
IN THE ROAD ...

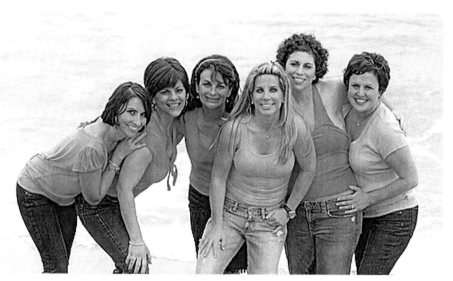

www.alumpintheroad.com

JUST a LUMP IN THE ROAD ...

✦

Reflections of young breast cancer survivors

Six young women and their families talk candidly about their battles with breast cancer, sharing information and insight known only to those who have experienced it. Each story has a unique perspective as diverse as the women themselves.

Written by:
Debbie Leifert
Gina Castronovo
Dr. Tamara Brennan
Jackie Ehrlich
Cindy Goldberg
Donna Palmisciano

iUniverse, Inc.
New York Bloomington Shanghai

JUST a LUMP IN THE ROAD ...

Reflections of young breast cancer survivors

iUniverse books may be ordered through booksellers or by contacting:

iUniverse
1663 Liberty Drive
Bloomington, IN 47403
www.iuniverse.com
1-800-Authors (1-800-288-4677)

Because of the dynamic nature of the Internet, any Web addresses or links contained in this book may have changed since publication and may no longer be valid.

The views expressed in this work are solely those of the author and do not necessarily reflect the views of the publisher, and the publisher hereby disclaims any responsibility for them.

ISBN: 978-0-595-45926-1 (pbk)
ISBN: 978-0-595-70806-2 (cloth)
ISBN: 978-0-595-90226-2 (ebk)

Printed in the United States of America

DEDICATION

This book is dedicated to all women and their families battling breast cancer. May they find strength, courage and support through our words. And to Darci McNally; without you there would be no us.

To my husband, Doug, for his unwavering support and love. To my very special boys, Isaac and Ethan for brightening every single one of my days. To my parents for being there for us, everyday. Lee, David, Syd and Jules my strength and example of the true meaning of human compassion. Stephanie, Adam, Alana and Emily my constant cheerleaders and shoulders to cry on. Lori, Evan, Lindsay, Abby and Jason for ALWAYS being there without question. Thank you all for giving me a reason to battle breast cancer and supporting me every step of the way. I love you with all my heart, Debbie

All my love and gratitude to the following people who were in the trenches with me as I waged my war against cancer. To my husband Paul and children Nic and AJ for hanging in there with me. To my parents and in-laws for all their help. To Linda and Lauren for disrupting their lives while attending to mine. To my sister and brothers who understood. To Sharilyn for her willingness to share. To my legion of friends, too many to name, who became chefs and chauffeurs and everything in between. To all the doctors and health care professionals who cared for my body and to everyone who prayed for me, sending me positive energy, you lifted my soul. I am truly humbled by your love. I would also like to thank all the cancer researchers and fund raisers who have devoted their lives to finding a cure. Finally, to all the women who have come before me, who participated in drug trials and have given me hope for the future. Gina

I would like to dedicate this book to my family and friends for their constant support and love during my battle against breast cancer. Tim, my loving and strong husband, thank you for being my rock through it all. Shauna, you are my inspiration! Mom and dad, thank you for your unending love and support. I could not have gone through this with out you. Love, Tamara.

To my wonderful husband, David, thank you for ALWAYS supporting me. To my children, Steven, Bradley and Michelle, I am so proud of all of you and you mean the world to me. Thank you, David and Joann Applebaum for being with me and getting everything done in record time. To "uncle" for being my cheerleader, thank you for your strength and encouragement. I love you, Jackie.

To my "inner circle" of family and friends Mom, Frank, Nanny, Aunt Debs, Robin, Karyn, Lisa, Richie, Sherri, Jill, Wendy, Amy (exotic flower), Helen, the 'mules, Dominique/Karen (treatment goddesses), the Karzen/Mandel clans and my incredibly expanding theatre family (especially Kat and Mini Me)—I love you! Thank you for loving, laughing, crying, and supporting me on this journey. To my doctors—Thank you for being exactly who you are and for doing what you do. To all the secret angels who appeared and offered the "kindness of strangers" I am eternally grateful and thankful. To Wayne, welcome to this wonderful new world and thank you for coming into my life. To the BBF's—my newest sisters—I love you and am blessed to have found you. Love, love, love. Mwah, Mwah, Mwah. Cindy

This book is dedicated to all the people who profoundly touched my life during such a life defining experience. I was blindsided with a cancer diagnosis at a pivotal time in my life. My hope is that this book will enrich all young women walking down the path that I've traveled and help them realize that breast cancer is *just a lump in the road*. I want to thank God for the gift of life! My mom, dad, sister and brothers for consistently being there for me, Patrick, my angel and biggest supporter, all of the wonderful heroes in our support group, my close girlfriends, my boss Steve and our fearless leader, Darci. Donna

Contents

ACKNOWLEDGMENTS

JUST a LUMP IN THE ROAD ... was made possible through the generosity and cooperation of many friends and associates who we would like to acknowledge. The six of us would like to thank Darci McNally always, Phyllis Steinberg for her direction, Susan Lantham for sharing her expertise in Lymphedema, Alisha Stein for her insight and compassion, Doctors Benda, Dudak, Porterfield, Lubetkin, Rosenthal and Vogel for lending their expertise to our project, Sherry Ferrante Photography for her wonderful pictures, Michelle Pallack of the John Michelle Salon for helping us feel beautiful, Michelle Joy for her countless hours editing and valuable input, our webmaster, Paras Wadehra (ParasWadehra@yahoo.com) for designing our incredible website www.alumpintheroad.com, Frank Marchone for the use of his antique Cadillac, John M. Cappeller, Jr. for his legal guidance, Chris Dardet at DardetPR for helping us to share our stories, Boca Raton Community Hospital for providing the space for our support group to meet and the Hillsboro Club for providing the backdrop for our photographs. Along with your assistance, we have turned our stories from the road into a visitors guide.

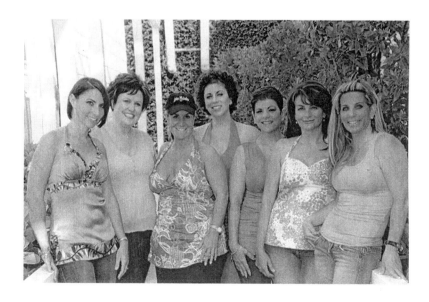

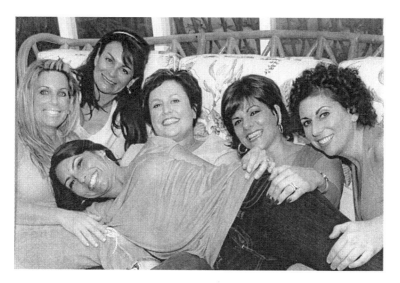

PREFACE

The purpose of this book is to inform, empower, enlighten and uplift the spirit of young women who are faced with a breast cancer diagnosis and treatment decisions. The manuscript tries to conquer the unique fears and concerns of a younger woman as she battles for her life with breast cancer. It was written by breast cancer survivors to give women faced with the disease the knowledge that they are not alone in this battle and that they can survive. It is also intended to provide support for all of the caregivers involved from spouses to bosses, children to babysitters, friends, boyfriends and significant others yet to come. This book will be an invaluable component of your support system and a shoulder to lean on during this difficult period.

FORWARD

The face of breast cancer is changing. Younger women are developing the disease. Although many of the concerns that a breast cancer patient faces are similar across the diagnosed population, some issues are unique to certain age groups. Many young women, who are single, newly married, and mothers of young children are developing the disease. It's not "our Mother's breast cancer" anymore—affecting mostly older women with more advanced diagnosis. As a result of breast cancer research, early detection now plays a major role in affording women a more favorable prognosis if diagnosed with breast cancer. It has also had a profound impact on the psychosocial field of medicine.

As the director of Multimodality Oncology Care at Lynn Cancer Institute, I started a support program for young women that were diagnosed with breast cancer. This support group far surpassed any expectations that I had hoped to fulfill. As the oncology social worker in our Breast Multimodality Clinic, I see all of the newly diagnosed patients for an initial interview and consult. My cancer center was already hosting breast cancer support groups, but the demographics did not meet or match the needs of younger women.

The criterion for this new program was a recent diagnosis of breast cancer for women under the age of 50. The group was scheduled to meet once a month. After the first meeting, I could already see it was the beginning of something much larger. The demographic diversity of these women was vast in terms of their race, religion, socioeconomic status, marital status and children status. Still, the "connection" was intense. These women began meeting outside the support group a second time each month on their own for dinner, socialization and support. The phone tree grew, as well as their support for one another. They developed a bond that can only be described as sisterhood. They chose to attend each others chemotherapy appointments, wig appointment and reconstruction appointments.

On a regular basis I witnessed the "pay it forward" mentality which I believe was the impetus for writing this book. As the women got further along in their own personal journeys they became the mentor for the new women in the group helping them through the challenges. I believe this book is an opportunity for all young women diagnosed with breast cancer that can not come to our group to benefit from the support and wisdom of our sisterhood.

Darci McNally, LCSW

Director of Multimodality Oncology care and the site specific oncology social worker for the Breast Multimodality Clinic at the Lynn Cancer Institute at Boca Raton Community Hospital in Boca Raton, Florida. Darci has been in the field of PsychoOncology for 12 years. Her strong passion for the breast cancer population has shifted the majority of her practice to breast only. She has seen many advances in all aspects of breast cancer over the span of her career, which is one of the reasons she finds it so rewarding.

CHAPTER ONE

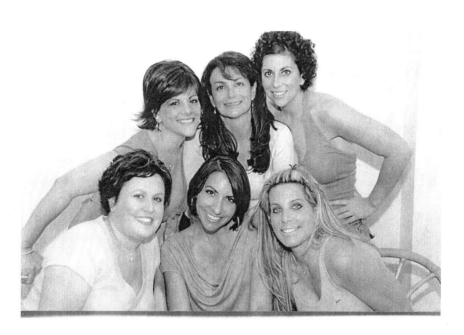

THE SURVIVORS:
LET THE JOURNEY BEGIN

"I joined a support group that was suggested to me by my doctors. I felt an instant connection and sense of belonging to other women in the group. As bizarre as the idea of this sounds, this diverse group of women have ended up becoming my good friends that I know will always be a part of my life."

—Jackie

Our journey began, much like that of every other woman diagnosed with breast cancer: shock, disbelief and the question "how could this happen to me?" The difference was that we were all under the age of 43. Our group was comprised of a newlywed, two singles and three married mothers.

Today, approximately one in eight women is diagnosed with breast cancer. Currently there are more than 250,000 survivors in the United States under the age of 45. These women are daughters, wives and mothers whose illnesses and subsequent treatments affect their entire families. They face issues unique to our age group.

We found each other through a support group and realized how comforting it is to have a friend who knows exactly how you are feeling. We shared information and gave insight to one another because we were all walking in the same shoes. As the bond that we felt for each other and our friendships grew, the realization of how lucky we were to have each other was evident.

Welcome to our club, our sisterhood, our family. As each of us reflects on our journey, secrets are divulged and modesty is not an issue. Each story is as diverse and unique as each one of us. We discuss dating and mastectomies, children and mortality, treatment and hair loss, caring for each other and our caregivers. We are hoping to give a voice to the young survivor and provide validation and encouragement to anyone battling this disease.

Let us wage this battle with you. Welcome. Welcome to our club.

DEBBIE LEIFERT
AGE AT DIAGNOSIS: 37
FAMILY HISTORY: None
BIOPSY RESULTS:
Infiltrating poorly differentiated Ductal Carcinoma
Stage II, Tumor size: 1.7 cm
Sentinel Nodes: 2 positive of 3
Auxiliary: 1 positive of 4
Estrogen Receptors (ER): Positive
Progesterone Receptors (PR): Positive
HER2Neu: Negative
THERAPY:
Lumpectomy
Chemotherapy
Triptorelin intramuscularly every 28 days for 10 months leading up to
Oophorectomy
Radiation Therapy
Tamoxifen Hormonal Therapy
RESEARCH STUDIES:
A Phase II Feasibility Trial Incorporating Bevacizumab (Avastin) into
Dose Dense Doxorubicin and Cyclophosphamide followed by Paclitaxel
in Patients with Lymph Node Positive Breast Cancer.
A Phase III Trial Evaluating the Role of Exemestane Plus GnRH Analogue
as Adjuvant Therapy for Premenopausal Women with endocrine Responsive Breast Cancer.

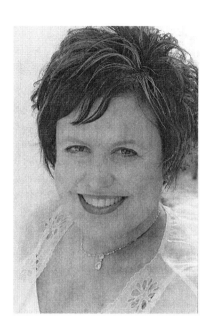

DEBBIE LEIFERT

Debbie was born in Indianapolis, IN and moved to South Florida when she was a teenager. She attended the University of Florida, earned a Master's Degree in Early Childhood Education and was a teacher for 10 years. She has been married for eight years and is the mother of two handsome young boys, ages five and seven. She enjoys traveling and spending time with her family and friends. Her favorite place to vacation is in the White Mountains of New Hampshire.

She was diagnosed at the age of 37. She discovered a small lump in her breast while in the shower. Although Debbie did not have a family history of breast cancer, she called her OBGYN that day and asked to be seen. Her proactive behavior is something she feels is important to share with other women. She was given an excellent prognosis because her breast cancer was detected early. It was a very aggressive fast growing cancer. Had she waited until her next yearly checkup or her mammogram that wasn't required to take place until she was 40, her prognosis would have been very different.

Debbie is an active member of her community and a dedicated supporter of raising the awareness of breast cancer and educating others.

GINA CASTRONOVO

AGE AT DIAGNOSIS: 42

FAMILY HISTORY: A Great Aunt that was diagnosed late in life.

BIOPSY RESULTS:

Infiltrating extensive ductal carcinoma, in-situ

Stage III Comedo type, high grade,

Tumor sizes: 5 x 7 cm and two additional smaller tumors

Lymph Nodes: Sentinel node biopsy: 2 of 4 positive

Estrogen Receptors (ER): Negative

Progesterone Receptors (PR): Negative

HER2Neu: Positive

THERAPY:

Bilateral Mastectomy with Reconstruction

Chemotherapy

Herceptin

Radiation Therapy

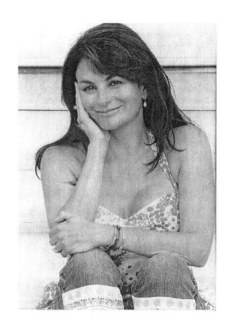

GINA CASTRONOVO

A bit of a nomad, Gina was born in Chicago but spent most of her youth in Boca Raton, FL. There she enjoyed a happy, active childhood as the oldest of five children. She attended several colleges and universities, earning two degrees. After which, Gina spent a number of years in the music business booking bands, buying talent and working for a concert promoter. Eventually, she became an instructor and administrator at the Art Institute of Ft. Lauderdale. Gina has been married since 1996 to a popular radio and television host. She has two children and is a stay at home Mom. She loves to travel with her family and to go boating. Some of their favorite destinations are the Bahamas, the northeastern United States and Italy.

Gina was always diligent about her yearly mammograms and check ups, although the most that had ever been revealed was a "dense breast" diagnosis. Then, one morning she awoke with one breast that was very swollen. Immediately she sought attention. That would be the beginning of her journey. Gina was only 42 years old.

Together Gina and her husband Paul seek to raise awareness and to educate people about breast cancer. Gina continues today to be a strong voice for the cause, and most certainly, always will be.

TAMARA BRENNAN

AGE AT DIAGNOSIS: 31

FAMILY HISTORY: My sister at age 33 was diagnosed one month before me.

BIOPSY RESULTS:

Two separate infiltrating ductal carcinoma

Stage I

Tumor sizes: 1.6 cm and 0.8 cm

Lymph Nodes: Left and right side all were negative

Estrogen Receptors (ER): Positive

Progesterone Receptors (PR): Positive

HER2Neu: Positive

THERAPY:

Bilateral Mastectomy with Reconstruction

Chemotherapy Treatment

Herceptin Treatments

Tamoxifen Hormonal Therapy

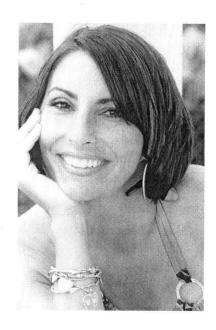

TAMARA BRENNAN

Tamara was born in Lancing, MI, but grew up in Arkansas. She earned a degree in Biology from the University of Central Arkansas and then graduated from Louisiana State School of Veterinary Medicine in 2002. She has lived in Florida for five years and is currently an associate veterinarian at a practice in her community. She has been married for two years to the love of her life. They have two dogs and two cats that are a part of the family. Tamara enjoys mountain biking, scuba diving, running, working out, triathlon sprints, boogie boarding and reading romance novels.

Shortly after Tamara's wedding, she received the heartbreaking news that her older sister, Shauna, had been diagnosed with breast cancer, Tamara immediately went for a mammogram. Their diagnoses ended up being one month apart. Tamara was 31 years old, her sister age 33. They had no family history of breast cancer and were instantly bonded in a way they could have never imagined. Across the miles, Shauna lived in Texas, and with several phone calls a day, they endured. They shared and supported each other every step of the way.

Now Tamara and Shauna are participating in a sister study research project. They continue to support each other and hope for a future with a cure for breast cancer.

JACKIE EHRLICH
AGE AT DIAGNOSIS: 42
FAMILY HISTORY: None
BIOPSY RESULTS:
Stage I
Tumor size: 1.8 cm X 1.5 cm
Lymph Nodes: Sentinel Node had some cancer cells
Estrogen Receptors (ER): Positive
Progesterone Receptors (PR): Positive
HER2Neu: Positive
THERAPY:
Bilateral Mastectomy with Reconstruction
Chemotherapy
Herceptin
Tamoxifen Hormonal Therapy

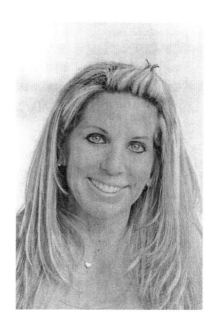

JACKIE EHRLICH

Jackie met the love of her life 25 years ago in Silver Springs, MD. She has three beautiful children, two boys and a girl. After the birth of her daughter her family relocated to Florida. She and her husband are entrepreneurs of a very successful business in the food industry. They have never shied away from a challenge and battling breast cancer was no different. Jackie runs everyday and enjoys exercise. If you ask her what she is passionate about, the answer is easy, it is her family.

Jackie's fight against breast cancer began with a self breast exam. At the age of 42, she found a lump in her breast. She had no family history of breast cancer, but the idea of how this could impact her children was always in the forefront of her mind.

Jackie was a major part of the glue that held the support group together. Her openness and genuine willingness to help others kept the group strong. Today, she is still contacted daily by newly diagnosed women for support. She has become a match-maker of sorts, connecting women with other women around the same stage of their treatment. She is making a difference, literally, one person at a time.

CINDY GOLDBERG

AGE AT DIAGNOSIS: 36

FAMILY HISTORY: BRCA 1 from my father's side of the family. Aunt diagnosed with breast cancer at 35 years old. She is still living.

BIOPSY RESULTS: No biopsy was taken; initial lump was thought to be a cyst. The pathology report diagnosed cancer.

Infiltrating poorly differentiated ductal carcinoma

Stage II

Tumor sizes: approximately 1.9 cm

Lymph Nodes: None

Estrogen Receptors (ER): Negative

Progesterone Receptors (PR): Negative

HER2: Negative

THERAPY:

Bilateral Mastectomy with Reconstruction—Becker Implant

Chemotherapy

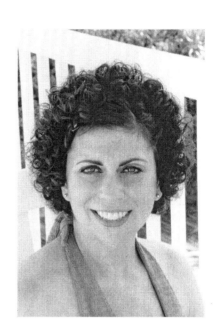

CINDY GOLDBERG

Born in the suburbs of Chicago, Cindy lived in Deerfield, IL until Junior High School when her family moved to Littleton, CO. The youngest of three girls, Cindy attended the University of Michigan where she double majored in Political Science and Communications. Cindy spent twelve years working for MCI, splitting her time between Sales and Marketing. She lived in Chicago, the D.C. metro area, and Tampa before settling in South Florida in the year 2000.

Currently the Marketing Manager for a Healthcare Communications Company, Cindy was single during her diagnosis and treatment. She is also very active in local area theatre. In addition, Cindy is an avid traveler, photographer and painter.

Cindy discovered a lump while performing a monthly self breast exam and was told it was a cyst. Only after it was removed did the pathology reveal it was cancer. Cindy was 36 years old when she began her cancer journey.

DONNA PALMISCIANO
AGE AT DIAGNOSIS: 40
FAMILY HISTORY: None
BIOPSY RESULTS:
Infiltrating ductal carcinoma
Tumor sizes: 3.8 cm, 0.7 cm and 0.4 cm
Lymph Nodes: Left and right side sentinel nodes were all negative
Estrogen Receptors (ER): Positive
Progesterone Receptors (PR): Positive
HER2Neu: Negative
THERAPY:
Bilateral Mastectomy with Reconstruction
Chemotherapy
Radiation Therapy
Hormonal Therapy

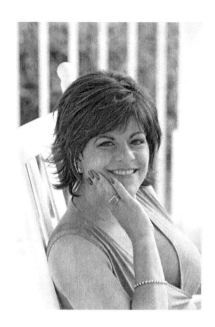

DONNA PALMISCIANO

Donna was born in Stony Brook, L.I., New York and has moved around throughout her childhood. Finally, her parents settled in South Florida when she was eleven and hasn't left since. She attended the University of Florida's school of Architecture and received a bachelor's degree in Interior Design. Donna currently enjoys working for an architectural firm and specializes in commercial design.

Donna, at age 40, was shocked to find out she had breast cancer while following the protocols for breast reduction surgery. Her cancer was detected on the mandatory mammogram and ultrasound required before a breast reduction can be performed.

She has a true passion for the beauty of nature, spending time outdoors and loves animals. With her free time, Donna loves to travel and try new experiences. She has always treasured her close friends and family and enjoys spending time with them whenever possible. Being involved in the community has always been important to her and she will go out of her way to help others.

As you read on, you will get to know each of us more intimately. Our hope is that we will help other young women diagnosed with breast cancer to know that they are not alone, that we all share many of the same fears and struggles, worries and concerns. As we talk about our journeys with breast cancer, we hope you will find comfort in our words. Use this book as a guide, as a shoulder to lean on, as a reference for what the next step might be. Allow us to help you as we helped each other.

CHAPTER TWO

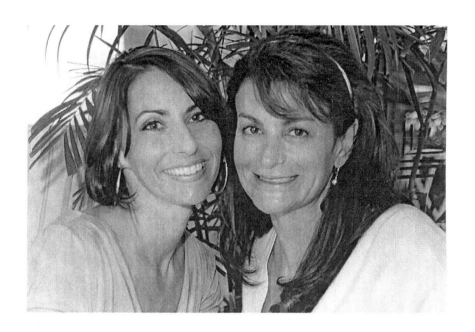

EMPOWERMENT: TAKING CONTROL

"The moment I got back in the car I realized that I needed to start taking control of the diagnosis, of the game plan. This was my body, my life and I needed to be sure I was making the right decisions for me. That night I was going to be with my family and friends—surrounded by their love and support. Tomorrow, I would start figuring out my plan.

—Cindy

As we began our journeys, everything seemed very surreal. We were being bombarded with important information and being asked to make life changing decisions. We had to make medical decisions that we had no background knowledge in and did not feel qualified to make. We had to decide whether or not to get a second opinion and what to do with that information. We had to choose one major surgery or another and even how often and when to have our treatments. All the while, we tried to maintain a sense of normalcy for our young children, husbands or significant others. The doctor appointments were numerous and the phone calls and discussions were exhausting. Friends and family members were all concerned and wanted information. Non medical "advice" was dished out whether it was wanted or not.

As each of us joined the support group, we each felt as if the roller coaster slowed down a little. With the guidance of our outstanding facilitator, Darci, we were able to speak, learn and make sense of what the doctors were asking of us. We were all on the same page, speaking the same language.

You will have to decide which surgery to have, which treatment course to take and how often, etc. This is it. This is the time in your life when you need to bring your A Game, as they say, and we are here to help. The following is meant to inspire, encourage and empower you. Take charge of your diagnosis and your journey. Take it one day, or one minute at a time if you need to, but become an active participant in your fight against breast cancer. You can do it, we believe in you.

TAMARA

I had cancer and I wanted it out right away. Yet, I knew that some of my decisions would affect the rest of my life. Being a physician and communicating with doctors on a daily basis, I know that unfortunately some doctors are better than others. I knew that I didn't have to just nod my head and go along with everything they were saying. I knew I had to be in control, as difficult as that was, in such a stressful situation. I relied heavily on my common sense and my medical background to make sure that what they were saying was logical. I asked every question I could think of concerning my course of treatment. I tried not to just think in the short term, but of the big picture as well. I asked how often the doctors had dealt with young women. I looked at the overall treatment plan with respect to how to organize it best for me, to become the best advocate for myself.

GINA

At the time of my diagnosis, I had recently joined the ranks of women in their 40's and was settling in nicely. Both my children were now off to school. My husband's career put us in the public eye, a somewhat demanding but always interesting place to be. I was comfortable in my skin, confident with my social skills and grateful for my education. I could carry on a conversation with an NFL football coach or a famous actor. We enjoyed private functions, great trips, yachts, tickets to all the best events, and great tables at restaurants. For the most part it was great to be me. I was empowered, or so I thought.

Then, like a lightning strike, I received the diagnosis of Stage III breast cancer. I realized all my perceived power was just a fallacy. I felt alone, challenged, overwhelmed and unprepared. My social circle was replaced with a new inner circle of doctors, nurses, technicians, office personal and counselors. My education did little to prepare me for the decisions I would need to make. I did not speak the language of cancer, but I would become a quick study. Initially, my husband and loved ones did the internet research and followed me to a myriad of doctor's appointments. They asked questions and took notes while I was too overwhelmed to remember what was being said. Perhaps my mind was trying to protect me from a complete mental meltdown. Slowly, I began to understand why people often referred to cancer survivors as warriors, heck I would have to fight for my life. I also had to protect myself from those that might stand in the way of victory.

In the beginning, tears flowed every morning as I awoke to the realization that it wasn't just a nightmare. I had cancer. It was my life. The three weeks that followed my diagnosis were a whirlwind. I had three biopsies and countless scans. My case was presented at tumor board and I went to a multi modality clinic. I got a second opinion which was arranged by friends. I had a sentinel node biopsy surgery and a port inserted into my arm. I assembled a team of doctors and arranged to have chemotherapy. I also hosted my best friend's wedding reception at my house. We broke the news to the children. And to wrap it up, I accompanied my husband on a radio station trip to the Bahamas with 650 listeners who, at the time were unaware of my situation.

It was now October, breast cancer awareness month, a difficult time for newly diagnosed women. Stories and reminders of the disease are everywhere. My family and friends had returned to their routines. For me however, the doctor's appointments continued. My calendar was filled with appointments I'd rather not keep. I had not yet come to grips with my situation. Contributing to my exhaustion was the fact that I had recently suffered a horrible rib and sternum injury and had just finished almost a year of physical therapy four months earlier. One morning, my schedule brought me to the office of Dr. Louise Morrell. I was still sporting the "deer in the headlights" look. I told her I wasn't strong enough to fight. She looked at me empathetically and said, "Well then, we'll just have to drag you through it because dying is not an option." Her words hung in the air. I did not reach up to grab them that day, but at some point I did. I began to fight and the words "dying is not an option" became my battle cry (sometimes whimper).

Eventually, I began to feel empowered again. It was a slow burn fueled by knowledge and information. It was acquired through books and experience, encouraged and tended to by professionals. I knew what to expect at treatments. I was no longer intimidated by doctors or procedures. I became stronger with every gatekeeper I took on, be it insurance representatives or front desk personnel refusing me an appointment. I could walk into a chemotherapy room like it was a cocktail party. I even penned a little something that I sent to a few of the health care professionals who took care of me and so many of my new girlfriends.

I wrote: My wish is that I could wrap up the newly diagnosed breast cancer patients in yellow work tape with big black print that reads: CAUTION! HEALING IN PROGRESS. It would serve as a symbol to everyone entrusted with her care to proceed with caution; because just like a home that's being renovated, there's a lot of work being done under the façade. Try not to trip on the new wiring, or clog the plumbing. Please don't chip the plaster or leave your fingerprints in wet paint. And for heaven's sake, don't trample the new landscaping. Make sure when the job is all done, that this incredible woman will get a permanent certificate of occupancy for her newly renovated home.

DONNA

Upon learning that I had breast cancer, my first plan of action was to gather as much information as possible to see exactly what I was up against. Breast cancer does not run in my family and no one close to me had gone through it. I really didn't have much knowledge on the topic. Knowledge is power and I wanted to have as much control over this monster as possible. A facts and data kind of girl, I first went to the library and spent a few hours searching for books I thought would be helpful. I sure wish at the time, I was able to find a book about young women and breast cancer. I believe that everything happens for a reason. It is no coincidence that six of us young women wrote this book! I also looked on the Internet for all I could find out about breast cancer. To me, the information on the Internet was a little overwhelming and it was difficult to pinpoint exactly what I was looking for.

Shortly after my diagnosis, Darci, a social worker who works for the hospital where I was being treated, contacted me. She told me about the multi-modality clinic that is offered at the Lynn Cancer Center in Boca Raton, FL. I was able to meet with a radiation oncologist, genetic counselor, medical oncologist, radiation oncologist and my favorite social worker, Darci!, all in one morning at one location. It was a wonderful source of information and knowledge and very helpful with the formulation of a game plan for my fight. I was given recommendations from the Clinic for breast surgeons and reconstructive surgeons. I met with Dr. Colletta, my breast surgeon, and knew right away that I liked him and that he was the Doctor for me. I shopped around and interviewed four plastic surgeons before selecting one. Darci was very instrumental with helping to coordinate appointments and answer a lot of questions. Additionally, she invited me to join a support group for newly diagnosed young women. I was all for it and attended my first meeting several weeks before my surgery.

I met a great bunch of young women at my support group. One member, Cindy, took me under her wing and showed me the ropes. She directed me to get a flex folder to organize all the paperwork that would come flooding in. She was right! Today that folder is packed and overflowing with everything to do with my cancer. I took control of my situation by being organized and learning as much as I could about breast cancer. This gave me a sense of control over the cancer.

I feel being a single person and fighting breast cancer made it twice as hard on me emotionally. I felt very alone at times. There were times that I wished I was married, so that I would have someone who cared and loved me at my side for support. It would have been nice to have a partner help me through so many different situations that arose; lying in bed all day on my "sick days" during chemotherapy, times that I was in physical pain, or just too exhausted to work. I had to rally deep within myself to be strong and take care of myself. I had to pick my chin up and be an advocate for ME!! Yes, there were my mini pity-parties which lasted about five minutes and I would cry, and that was OK, it was part of the healing process. I didn't let myself stay in that place for too long; instead, I waged my battle with a positive outlook and humor.

DEBBIE

I feel it is important to remember is that it is your body and ultimately your decision how and whether you choose to proceed with treatment. You will hear the following from your doctors over and over, "This is what I would do, but you have to decide what is right for you". All the choices are yours, from something as minor as setting an appointment, to when to shave your head, to how often to have your chemotherapy treatments. So, I felt that if I was being handed that much power in my battle against breast cancer, I needed to be with doctors that felt it was important to educate me (and my family) along the way.

My husband and I immediately started researching the leading oncologists in the breast cancer field. We collected several names and made a decision to get three opinions and go from there. Each of the oncologists recommended basically the same procedures and course of treatment. The main difference I noticed was the manner in which the different doctors planned to communicate with my "team of doctors" and with us. It is important that your surgeon, oncologist, radiologist, general doctor, etc. are all up to date and communicate with each other about your ongoing care. I chose a teaching hospital, where I felt the most encouragement to be an active participant in my treatment. I was also greatly comforted by their desire to educate me about each decision, to explain to me what was happening and why. Once making the decision regarding which doctors would care for me and where, I felt ready to join my fight against breast cancer.

CINDY

I was lying on my bed talking on the phone to my best friend Lisa. I'd always performed self breast exams sporadically and this seemed like as good a time as any. I never expected to feel a lump in my right breast but there it was. It felt hard and kind of round. I said, "Hmm, I think I found a lump in my breast." She said,

"Really?" I said "Yeah, weird huh?" She said, "Well, you'd better get it checked out." I made an appointment the next day with my gynecologist, fully expecting it to be nothing.

My gynecologist checked out the lump and said "Yep, there's something definitely there but it feels like a cyst. I'll write you a prescription for a mammogram and an ultrasound and we'll check it out."

I walked into the clinic a little apprehensive but the techs were friendly and reassuring. The mammogram felt pretty much like I expected—cold and uncomfortable and the ultrasound was painless. Unfortunately, I was not able to get my results at that time and had to wait to hear from my doctor.

My gynecologist called three days later and said it looked like a cyst but to be safe, she suggested I meet with a surgeon to discuss options. I made the appointment for a few days later. The surgeon was a young woman—good since I figured she'd be knowledgeable and sympathetic to someone similar in age.

I started involving my mom at this point. I've always had an incredibly close relationship with her. On top of that, I have the kind of family that thinks nothing of attending doctor's appointments with each other and camping out if anybody is sick or in the hospital. So my mom and I met with the surgeon together. The surgeon reviewed my films and announced that they were "unimpressive"—a good thing, and most likely a cyst. However, she suggested removing it because the lump was a little large and in the "7 o'clock" position. I asked what this meant and she said to think of the breast like a clock. My lump was in the equivalent of "7 o'clock" on my breast.

I scheduled the appointment for the end of January. I've never been a big fan of hospitals and actually dread being put out with anesthetic. All seemed to go well. The surgeon actually stopped by the waiting room to tell my family that the procedure went well and it looked exactly like a cyst.

About a week later I went in for a check up—with Mom by my side once again for moral support. They told us to wait in the exam room for a few minutes. In retrospect, I do remember thinking it was strange that nobody asked me to put on a gown. When the doctor walked in she said "We got the pathology back and I'm sorry it's cancer." My mom and I looked at each other. My mom said "You're kidding right? You told us it was a cyst after the surgery." She said, "I'm so sorry, I wish I were."

At that moment, time stood still. I could barely breathe. Then awareness kicked in. I felt the path of my life alter irrevocably. In the blink of an eye, time went from frozen to warp speed. The surgeon started rattling off all these things that needed to be done asap: "I've made an appointment for you with a plastic surgeon. I'm sending you there now. I think we need to get in you within the next few weeks for a mastectomy with reconstruction. He's great, you'll like him."

After hearing the surgeon say "I'm sorry, it's cancer," I remember walking to the checkout desk. I was given directions to a nearby plastic surgeon's office and a reminder card with my mastectomy date as if it were just a dentist's appointment. We needed to get there in 20 minutes. I told my mom I needed to make some phone calls and I needed to do it in private.

I stood in the surgeon's parking lot for the next seven minutes, frantically calling my inner circle of friends knowing that I had to be at the plastic surgeon's office within the next 15 minutes. I remember saying that I needed a shot of tequila and thinking how funny that was since I'm not a drinker. The date was February 15, 2006.

On the ride to the plastic surgeon's office, my mind started reeling with questions. "Isn't this moving too fast? Is it smart to only have a single breast mastectomy? What about a lumpectomy? Why isn't anyone mentioning chemotherapy or radiation? How the hell did I get cancer? Why the hell did I get cancer? Is this really happening? Shouldn't I be exploring all my options? What about the breast cancer gene? How do I feel about the fact the surgeon misled my family after surgery? How can this be happening?"

We arrived at the plastic surgeon's office. He proceeded to tell us how he would perform the mastectomy and reconstruct the breast. When I started asking all the questions that were running through my brain he became very unresponsive. This was his area of expertise. He felt strongly about his plan and I was in too much shock to argue.

The moment I got back in the car, I realized I needed to take control of this situation. This was my body, my life. Nobody was going to tell me what to do unless I was 100% onboard.

I called my Gynecologist the next morning. I told her about my surgeon's diagnosis and shared my concerns regarding the quick mastectomy game plan. I said I felt like no one answered my questions.

My Gynecologist suggested that given my age, I might want to explore treatment options that combine surgery, chemotherapy and radiation. This was the first time that I would hear the term "Multi-Modality." Also, she suggested that I might want to checkout clinical trials and other practices dedicated to working strictly with breast cancer patients.

I decided that I needed to keep things organized. I needed to keep all my information, questions and reports in one place. I went out that afternoon and bought a journal and a tabbed portfolio that would allow me to quickly organize the mountain of information I anticipated collecting. I chose a bright, jewel encrusted journal and a bold colored portfolio. In my own way I was saying "Cancer, I'm not afraid of you and I am going to surround myself with happy, bright things in spite of you!"

I don't know what people did before the Internet. I Googled everything I could to find about breast cancer treatment in South Florida. I called various breast cancer support groups in my area including Y-me and the American Cancer Society. I also called my best friend Lisa and she already had tons of information for me that she collected from her mother-in-law—a breast cancer survivor.

A week later, I decided to go checkout the Boca Raton Community Hospital's Multi-Modality clinic. It was close by and it seemed to have a good reputation. I liked the idea of having a team fight this with me.

The program consisted of going to the hospital and meeting with a Genetic Counselor, an Oncologist, a Radiologist and a Social Worker. This team of specialists would independently review my results and discuss their areas of expertise with me. They would learn about me and then spend time answering my questions. Later, they would meet as a team, discuss my case and make recommendations for my treatment. The Oncologist would then meet with me, yet again, to discuss their suggestions for my treatment and get my feedback.

JACKIE

When I first learned that I had breast cancer, I was in shock. It felt as if I was watching it happen to somebody else. The phrases, I'm so young, I exercise everyday, I'm just too healthy, kept racing through my mind.

Unfortunately, women of all ages, shapes and sizes are at risk. Once the reality that I did have breast cancer started to sink in, I became scared. I felt out of control and I was afraid I was going to die. I didn't know who to turn to or what to do. My children were looking to me for answers, for a sign that our family was going to be ok. I knew I needed to pull myself together; but how?

With the help of my Oncologist, along with my family, I began gathering the courage and strength needed for my battle with breast cancer. I accepted the path that my life had led me down and began my journey.

You are now ready for battle. You are lining up a great team consisting of surgeons and oncologists, family and friends. You have some idea in mind about how you would like this to play out: what you expect and need from your doctors and support system. You are preparing for the onslaught of doctor appointments and information that is headed your way. Be strong in your convictions. Don't be afraid to ask questions or request copies of your records, films and scans at each appointment. Although at times it may not feel like it, you are in control. You are fighting for your life and dying is not an option. We believe in you.

THE MEDICAL TEAM:

OBSTETRICS AND GYNECOLOGY (OB/GYN)

David I. Lubetkin, MD, FACOG

David Lubetkin received his Bachelor's Degree from Johns Hopkins University and completed his Medical training at the Albert Einstein College of Medicine in 1992. He then completed his Residency in Obstetrics and Gynecology in 1996 at the North Shore University Hospital in New York. Currently he is in Private Practice in the fields of Obstetrics, Gynecology and Infertility.

Dr. Lubetkin is an active member of the local Medical Community. He has recently served as Chief of Staff of the West Boca Medical Center; as well as President of the Palm Beach County OB/GYN Society.

THOUGHTS ON BREAST CANCER IN WOMEN UNDER 45

I feel an important message for young women is that if you are going to get breast cancer, you want it detected as early as possible. The earlier the diagnosis is, the higher the chance for a cure.

Women need to be very diligent about their self breast examinations, annual breast exams with the gynecologist, and mammograms. They should ask their gynecologist to educate them on the correct way to perform a self breast exam and the correct time of the month to perform it. There are also many excellent websites that provide instructions and pictures. Such as the Susan Koman for the Cure website: www.Komen.org. Annual appointments should be kept to help maintain important baseline information regarding their gynecological health.

Many cases of breast cancer in young women are found on self exam. I wish more women would be extra conscientious about it. I have often said that Nike would have a great adjunct to their "just do it" advertising campaign by advocating self breast exams—women should "just do it".

A PERSONAL NOTE FROM THE DOCTOR

I chose this type of medicine because it provided me with a good mix of surgery and medical care with a relatively healthy patient population. I find it challenging and extremely rewarding.

SUPPORT/PSYCHOSOCIAL CARE

Darci McNally, LCSW

Darci McNally is a licensed clinical social worker. She received her Bachelor's Degree from the University of Massachusetts, Amherst and her Master's degree at Florida International University. She did a psychosocial training certification program at Memorial Sloan-Kettering in New York.

She has worked in the oncology setting for the last 12 years providing supportive counseling to patients and family members. She began her career at the Mount Sinai Comprehensive Cancer Center on Miami Beach. Currently she is the Director of Multimodality Oncology Care and Cancer Care Coordination at the Lynn Regional Cancer Center at Boca Raton Community Hospital. She facilitates stress management, psycho-educational and support groups. Currently her main focus is women's cancers specifically breast and gynecological, but does cover all varieties of cancer, wherever there is a need.

In addition, she is actively involved in the American Cancer Society and the Susan G. Komen for the Cure Foundation. She eagerly heads up fundraising efforts for these charities on behalf of the hospital and the community.

Darci makes her counseling and support services available to not only Boca Raton Community Hospital patients, but to anyone in the community that may require assistance.

THE ROLE OF SUPPORT/PSYCHOSOCIAL CARE IN RESPECT TO BREAST CANCER

Close to half of newly diagnosed breast cancer patients are found to have clinically significant emotional distress even before any treatment has begun (study Dec 2006 issue of Cancer). Mark Hegel, PhD from the Norris Cotton Cancer Center at Dartmouth Medical School conducted a psychiatric and functional screening of 236 newly diagnosed women with breast cancer and these were the findings: almost one in two women met clinically significant criteria for emotional distress or psychiatric disorder. The most common problem was moderate to severe emotional distress (41%). The most commonly reported source of distress was related to the cancer diagnosis (100%), followed by the uncertainty about treatment (96%) and concerns about physical problems (81%) Twenty one percent of the women met the criteria for psychiatric disorder including major depression (11%) and Post traumatic Stress disorder (10%). These women also demonstrated significant declines in daily functioning that were due to the emotional disorders. Treatment for their cancer had not yet begun.

The paragraph above is not intended to alarm. It IS intended to educate and validate that the emotional side of breast cancer is real and deserves to be attended to.

Each woman's breast cancer journey will be unique with respect to not only their type of breast cancer and their recommended treatments, but due to their own internal coping skills, family structure, financial situation, employment status and outside supports. It is imperative that treating this aspect of your cancer can be extremely important and often directly related to how you get through your journey. Most cancer programs will have some sort of support person built in to their program. This person often is an oncology social worker or a breast health navigator (RN) and is the starting point of helping to get your holistic treatment plan in order. These coordinators are often considered the center spoke of the wheel. They can assist in the tangible concrete chores of: helping with 2nd opinions, getting all your appointments in order, education, referral to support groups or counseling services, helping with financial and employment issues, referring you to wig and prosthetic vendors, linking you to outside community resources such as the American Cancer Society or the Susan G Komen For the Cure Foundation. If the coordinator is an oncology social worker their scope of practice will also include providing the direct supportive counseling. It is recommended that each breast cancer survivor align themselves with a coordinator as soon as they are diagnosed.

BENEFITS OF SUPPORT GROUP AND/OR COUNSELING

In my practice I have found support groups one of the most rewarding programs to work with and at the same time the most difficult to "recruit" for. What do people think when you mention support group? Often I get the response of "how does hearing about other people's problems help me?" or "I don't want to get more depressed" or "I have plenty of friends why would I need a support group?" I have found myself often in the role of a glorified sales person trying to explain the benefits of attending and participating in a support group.

Some benefits are:

• Receiving assistance coping with the emotional and practical aspects of the disease

- A confidential atmosphere to discuss the challenges of the illness with others who have experienced similar challenges

- Friendship, although no one ever wants to be a part of this new club or group, I have found many of my support group members have made new life long friendships from participating in a support group.

- Access to information about your "situation"

- A place to learn coping mechanisms

- Support for your sanity and confidence that you are not alone

- Assistance in dealing with family members, friends and work issues

Support groups are not for everyone and deciding to participate and finding the right one is not always easy to do. While any given group may or may not work for you personally, there are characteristics that make some groups more effective than others. Keep these in mind as you explore your own choices:

- A caring atmosphere and trust among the group members

- A comfortable mix of participants

- Clear structure and purpose; the group members should know why they are there and what will happen

- Agreement and understanding of group guidelines, including confidentiality

- A professional facilitator

THE WORKINGS OF A SUPPORT GROUP

Support groups have two main formats: those led by professional facilitators such as a nurse, social worker or psychologist; and those led by group members which are often called peer or self-help groups. Most cancer led support groups fall under the definition of "mutual aid". There is a professional facilitator who helps the group help one another by sharing experiences and giving input to one another while validating ones' concerns and feelings because they too are "walking in similar shoes". Often breast cancer support groups have two key components; an educational component where guest speakers are invited to come and lecture on breast cancer related topics and an emotional component where support and experiences are shared. There is broad agreement on what support groups offer.

HOW TO FIND A SUPPORT GROUP

If you are reading this book then presumably you are looking for a "site specific" support group for breast cancer. If you are receiving your care in a hospital based cancer center setting it may be easier to find a group. Most cancer programs will have a nurse or social worker assigned as a "navigator" that would be your point person to connect you with all the appropriate resources including a support group. If you are not connected with a comprehensive cancer program you can check newspapers listings or local telephone book. Often contacting a state or national organization devoted to breast cancer is an option; such as the American Cancer Society or Susan G Komen for the Cure Foundation. Finally there is the beloved internet which has been such a valuable tool for not only connecting people but as an informational resource as well.

Counseling on an individual basis is something that can be done in conjunction with attending a support group or instead of attending a support group. This will depend upon each individuals needs and how they are coping at the time. While some people are reluctant to seek counseling; studies show that having someone to talk to reduces stress and helps both mentally and physically. Counseling can provide emotional support to cancer patients (and their families) to better help understand their illness. Different types of counseling include individual, group, family and marital. Often within the context of a diagnosis the counseling is considered "solution focused", primarily focusing on how to cope and work through how the diagnosis and treatment is affecting the person's life. If you are at a comprehensive cancer program social workers should be available to provide this service. If you are at a private physician's office, ask the doctor or nurse who they recommend.

SPECIFIC NEEDS OF WOMEN UNDER 50 WITH BREAST CANCER

There have been a growing number of women under the age of 50 being diagnosed with breast cancer. Many of these women seem to have similar life situations and issues that were further complicated by their diagnosis of breast cancer. Managing careers, marriage or singlehood, children or still wanting them, body image and sexuality were all issues that needed to be attended to. Having a peer group of not only women with a similar disease, but at a similar point in life is an extremely powerful combination.

If this option is not available where you live, there are on-line breast chat rooms where you can still feel connected. Being young and diagnosed with a life threatening illness often feels like an oxymoron. Breast cancer is not a death sentence, but it can feel that way and can feel even more threatening when you are young.

A PERSONAL NOTE FROM THE SOCIAL WORKER

You are not an anomaly. It is not why me? Rather, why not you, or me or anyone? The good news is the technology for detection and treatment is has advanced greatly over the past decade and continues to do so as we speak. Get educated, get support and keep on living. You can't control the fact that you got cancer, but you can control how much it controls your life!!

BREAST SURGEON

Marla Weissler Dudak, MD

Dr. Marla Dudak completed her Medical School training at Duke University, School of Medicine in 1995. She then went home to Miami and completed a five year general surgery residency at Jackson Memorial Hospital at the University of Miami. She did a one year fellowship in breast disease at University of Texas Southwestern in Dallas. At the time, there were only about six to eight funded breast fellowship programs. Cancer centers like Sloan Kettering were rare. The now reclaimed Moffitt Center in Tampa and MD Anderson in Houston did not have funded breast programs. Today there are over 25 funded breast fellowship programs in the United States.

She is currently in private practice as a solo practitioner. She treats men and women with breast problems only. Roughly 20% of her practice is cancer related. The other common problems she sees are related to breast pain, abnormal mammograms, benign lumps, and men and women with a family history of breast and ovarian cancer. She has two ultrasound machines in her office and does her own core biopsies, cryoablation of benign tumors, genetic counseling for high risk women and cyst aspirations.

THE ROLE OF A BREAST SURGEON IN BREAST CANCER TREATMENT

Breast cancer is a disease that requires all modalities to get the best results. This includes the surgeon, medical oncologist, radiation oncologist, geneticist, plastic surgeon, radiologist and pathologist. I feel in this community, the surgeon acts as the quarterback of the team. Passing the ball off when it is necessary, but always keeping track of how the game is going.

As a surgeon, cutting the cancer out is my primary role. I believe a lot of thought should go into what type of surgery is performed, the location of the scar, and if oncoplastic techniques should be employed.

THOUGHTS ON THE FUTURE OF BREAST CANCER TREATMENT

I hope that general surgeons come up to speed in how to take care of breast cancer patients. I hope that women have access to second opinions and immediate reconstruction in an era of dwindling reimbursement. I hope that MRI will continue to improve their sensitivity and comes down in price such that it is the new screening tool of choice. I hope that all cancer centers will be modeled after ours, in that a tumor board/multimodality is available to all new cancer patients. I hope that we find new targeted therapies such that even "triple negatives" have something in their armamentarium.

GREATEST ACHIEVEMENTS TO DATE FOR YOUNG WOMEN WITH A BREAST CANCER DIAGNOSIS

There have been amazing achievements in imaging, reconstruction, and less mutilating surgeries. Sentinel lymph node biopsies, partial breast irradiation, and lumpectomies have changed breast cancer treatment dramatically in the last 20 years. For premenopausal women in particular, the ability of MRI to see through dense breasts is awesome.

A PERSONAL NOTE FROM THE DOCTOR:

I became a breast surgeon for no dramatic reason. I love the constantly evolving aspect of breast cancer. I love my patients. I love making a difference.

DR. LEE PORTERFIELD, M.D., F.A.C.S.
PERSONAL REFLECTIONS ABOUT SURGICAL ISSUES FOR
YOUNG BREAST CANCER PATIENTS

Although the practice of surgical oncology/breast surgery is gratifying, there is nothing more difficult or more challenging than telling a young woman that she has cancer of the breast. The news is difficult to give to a woman of any age, but after all these years; I have still not found the right way to say it to a young patient. "The pathologist sees worrisome cells." "They see abnormal cells." "We see suspicious cells." I have finally decided that there is no right way to tell her. How could there be? It just isn't right.

Eventually though, I manage to get it out: "We have the result of your biopsy. The pathologist sees cancer cells." Then I pause ... out of respect and necessity. Her world has just stopped. I can't pause for too long, though, or I will get caught up in her pain and confusion, and then not be able to do my job. Then we go on, one critical step at a time, rebuilding her hopes and her dreams that for one earth-shattering moment, she incorrectly thought she might have to give up.

CHAPTER THREE

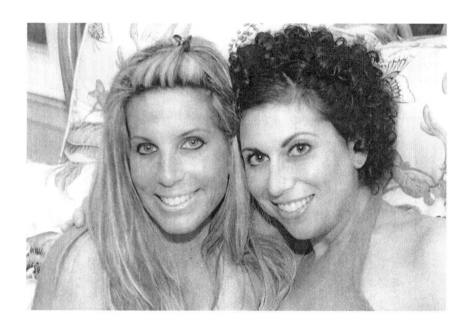

SURGERY:
GETTING IT OFF YOUR CHEST

"Having read many articles and books written by cancer survivors, both women and men, I realized that all cancer survivors share many of the same emotions and challenges. We often describe our journeys with identical words. But for those diagnosed with breast cancer, we are set apart by the mastectomy. The disfigurement is undeniable. It is a physical and mental hurdle that we must somehow get over."

—Gina

When you are diagnosed with breast cancer, the first important decision is usually what kind of surgery to have; a lumpectomy or a mastectomy. Due to the latest advances in breast cancer research and the ability to be able to find breast cancer in women at a much earlier stage, women now have more choices. With choices come consequences. For all of us it was an agonizing question that was researched thoroughly, talked about repeatedly and mulled over extensively even after the surgery was complete.

Our best advice is that you have to decide what feels right for you. Each breast cancer diagnosis is different, with different characteristics, and every woman has unique and individual needs. Decide what is going to be the most beneficial for your health, both physically and emotionally and go from there.

As you read on, we hope that we will be able to answer some of the hundreds of questions that are swirling around in your head. Questions you find difficult to discuss with others who have not experienced what you are going through. One in seven women will be diagnosed with breast cancer. You are not alone.

LUMPECTOMY VS. MASTECTOMY

"... the question was, "What about the other side?"

—*Tamara*

GINA

The large size of my tumor necessitated a mastectomy. I did, however have to choose between a single or double mastectomy. For me, the choice was simple. I wanted to eliminate the source of my cancer, all my breast tissue. My own body had betrayed me and who was to say it wouldn't happen again. Like toxic friends, they both would have to go. One was making me sick and the other would make me sick with worry.

Although the decision was made very quickly, the surgery would not happen for five months. The doctors had decided at a meeting called "tumor board" that the best treatment for me would be neo-adjuvant chemotherapy. *Neo-adjuvant* was another one of those strange words in the vast new language I was learning. Basically, it meant that I would have chemotherapy first to shrink my large tumor and then the surgeons would take it out. Trying not to become overwhelmed by the thought of my impending mastectomy was difficult. The fear of how it would look and feel terrified me, as I carried around the killer 5 X 7 cm. tumor waiting for it to shrink.

But shrink it did and by the time my surgery rolled around, I was ready to say goodbye to the girls. I felt worse for my husband than I did for myself. Although he never said it, he would miss them terribly. We had a going away party for the double D's. The evening involved lingerie and a lot of wine. We would send them off in style and try not to dwell in the past.

To ease my pre-surgery anxiety, I did however bring something from my old life to the procedure. It was a silly pedicure I originally got prior to the birth of my second son-sort of a Spring look with a different pastel color on each toe. The "Easter Egg Pedi" turned out to be quite a hit. I thought "why not do it again and give everyone in the Operating Room something to talk about.?" I continued the ritual with each of my subsequent surgeries. So, while some women wore lipstick to their mastectomies, I chose Easter egg toes.

Mastectomies are customized for each patient depending on many factors. My surgery involved a modified radical mastectomy on the cancer side. All the tissue and lymph nodes were taken. Most of the skin was taken as well. On the other side, a simple mastectomy was performed. Both nipples were also removed. I chose to begin reconstruction immediately and the surgery took approximately five hours. When I awoke I was bandaged and three freaky little tubes with balls on the ends were sticking out of the bandages. They were drains placed there to collect fluid. The drains were uncomfortable and nerve-racking, especially in the shower. I would hang them around my neck using safety pins and an old head band. I found sweat pants with pockets to be very helpful because I could tuck them in without much effort. My plastic surgeon removed the drains after 11 days. My recovery took about six weeks. During that time it was important to do wall walking exercises that my surgeon showed me to maintain the mobility in my arms. As for my mental recovery, that is still a work in progress.

JACKIE

My decision resulted in having a double mastectomy. I thought I had asked all the right questions and gathered enough information. Still, there were some very important things that I feel I didn't know or "wasn't able to hear" at the time when I was making that decision. Valuable information that I feel compelled to share with others that are going through a similar experience.

A double mastectomy doesn't automatically mean that you will not have to do chemotherapy or radiation. You should also keep in mind that you will be losing a part of your body, which many women equate with their sexuality. Even if you choose to do a reconstruction procedure, your reconstructed breasts will not have nerve endings or nipples. You may choose to have nipples drawn on using a tattoo process or by using skin from another area of your body. This usually takes place at the end of the reconstruction process and usually after treatment is over. It is also important to note that the reconstruction process takes a very long time. It involves many different steps, most of which require time for your body to heal between each one.

CINDY

After extensive research, I selected both my surgeon and plastic surgeon. I was surprised to learn that surgeons often prefer to work with certain plastic surgeons. So, in addition to your health insurance plan possibly restricting your options, it's possible that your surgeon may not want to work with your preferred plastic surgeon.

I chose my surgeon, because I appreciated the fact that when I met with him he told me ALL my options. He told me that ultimately the decision was mine. Unlike the first surgeon who told me exactly what would be done without considering my wishes, my selected surgeon was ready to do what I wanted.

I had taken the genetic test to see if I was a carrier of the BRCA Cancer gene but would not have the results for a few weeks. Even without knowing the results, I decided to go with a double mastectomy. Even though there was no sign of cancer in my left breast, I had read enough to learn that many young women who are diagnosed with Breast Cancer and only remove one breast or elect a lumpectomy, often have a recurrence within five years. Also, based on the genetic counseling I had received when I took the BRCA test, I knew I was at high risk having a relative with Breast Cancer and being an Ashkenazi Jew. For me, I was only going through this once. In addition, being 36 years old, I was still pretty proud of my breasts and wanted them to look as similar as possible. If I was going to have one fabulous fake boob I might as well have two, perky, non-sagging firm breasts!

I chose my plastic surgeon because I heard he was one of the best in the area. He also invented a product called the Becker 50/50. The product acts as both an expander and a permanent implant thus eliminating the need to have a second surgery once the implant is in place.

DEBBIE

I had a lumpectomy initially because I had a mass in my left breast. I had received a "highly suspicious mass" diagnosis from a mammogram, ultrasound and fine needle biopsy. My doctors were concerned, too. At that point, I decided to book the next available surgery date (which was only a few days away) and have the mass removed.

There was still one more test that could have been performed that might have provided a more definite diagnosis, but at that point, I just wanted the "highly suspicious" growth out of my body. I didn't want worry about it one minute longer.

The surgery was successful and the breast surgeon had a pathologist attending the surgery test the mass and lymph nodes. They removed all of the cancer and three positive lymph nodes.

My next step was to meet with oncologists to determine a plan of action. All of this was done in a very short amount of time. Each oncologist suggested a similar treatment regimen.

Because I had such an aggressive form of breast cancer, the doctors recommended that treatment start as soon as possible. Having a mastectomy, in my case, would be a prophylactic measure. The information that I gathered during my chemotherapy and radiation treatments helped me make my decision about the mastectomy.

I had a PET/CT scan, which showed no other signs of cancer in my body. I had a breast MRI scan. I also had genetic counseling and testing, which concluded that I was not a carrier for either the BRCA 1 or BRCA 2 gene. I did not have a strong family history of breast cancer.

In addition, I consulted with several different oncologists, and their general consensus was that a lumpectomy plus chemotherapy, radiation and hormonal therapy gave me the same chance of reoccurrence as having a mastectomy.

I decided that I would prefer to take mammograms every six months for the rest of my life and forgo the mastectomy at that time.

DONNA

At the time of my diagnosis, I had just turned 40 and was recently divorced after a 13 year marriage. Newly single, I finally made the decision to have a breast reduction, something I had been considering for a long time. It was a decision that may have saved my life. While I was undergoing the pre-op testing for the surgery which included a mammogram and ultrasound, my tumor was identified. It was slow growing and hard to detect in my large dense breasts. Neither I nor my gynecologist had felt the lump during previous check-ups. The irony of situation did not go unnoticed. I was planning to have my breasts reduced, just not this way.

As women, we have the choice to do whatever we want with our bodies. Often the choice to have a lumpectomy or mastectomy is ours to make. Understandably, the surgeons we consult like to remain fairly neutral. I asked my surgeon, Dr. Colletta, "What would you recommend to your wife in this situation?" He told me he would tell her to get a double mastectomy. I was all for it, I made up my mind right then and there in the exam room. I felt that I was making the right decision and was ready to move forward.

My reasons for choosing to have a double mastectomy were complex. But, basically I was going for the best outcome after reconstruction. I wanted symmetry. More importantly, I wanted peace of mind. If I choose to keep my non cancerous breast, I would have to get mammograms every six months for the rest of my life. I just couldn't put myself through the mind games and the wondering. God forbid that it came back at a later time. I wound never want to go through the trauma all over again.

I asked my doctors to begin reconstruction at the time of my mastectomy because I didn't want to be totally flat-chested. I think that it would have been very unsettling and disturbing to see myself without some semblance of a breast. It would have been difficult to fit into my clothes and stuffing a breast prosthesis into my bra was not for me. It helped my self-esteem to have breast implants put in at the time of surgery.

TAMARA

My left breast had two lumps that were in different quadrants. This meant that the entire breast would need to be removed. So the question was, "What about the other side?" I didn't have to think about it at all. I went with my gut feeling which was to remove all breast tissue from my body. I am young with an aggressive form of cancer. I did not want to worry about the other side. I also wanted to have breasts that looked the same, even if they were both scarred. You have to look at the perks; this was a chance to have larger boobs! Also, I felt emotionally betrayed by my breasts. I had a very strong urge to get them off my body.

HARDEST PART ABOUT KNOWING YOU'RE GOING TO HAVE A MASTECTOMY

"Our little sisterhood has become quite famous for our bathroom meetings where breasts, scars, nipples and areolas are displayed, touched, and discussed like tomorrow's fashions. Leaving bald and fuzzy chicken heads taking a close second."

—Cindy

CINDY

One of the hardest things about knowing I was going to have a mastectomy was the unknown. I didn't know what to expect. I didn't know how to feel or how I would look after surgery and reconstruction.

What helped me the most was meeting other women who selected my same plastic surgeon. I was amazed how so many women in the "sisterhood" were willing to show me their breasts and let me feel them. Sounds crazy, right? But I am someone who needs facts to help deal with the unknown. So seeing and touching expanders, 50/50s, saline and silicone breasts helped me get my head around what I would become and experience.

Our little sisterhood has become quite famous for our bathroom meetings where breasts, scars, nipples and areolas are displayed, touched, and discussed like tomorrow's fashions. Displaying bald and fuzzy chicken heads takes a close second to seeing, touching and discussing our evolving new breasts.

TAMARA

Facing surgery and the impending recovery was overwhelming for me. I knew that I would have to take time off of work as a veterinarian. I was also dealing with the understanding that I would have two very odd shaped breasts for a while. Would I be strong enough? How would my husband deal with this? What about my friends and co-workers?

GINA

The hardest part about knowing I had to have a mastectomy was the horrifying thought of being disfigured. The memories of my mother's friends loomed large. (Those neighborhood ladies who had the surgery no one talked about.) The strange bras and prosthesis they had to wear back then. I knew medical science had come a long way, but I still worried about my appearance. How would I cope?

PREPARING FOR YOUR LUMPECTOMY OR MASTECTOMY SURGERY

"I was totally unprepared for the path my life would take as I was woke up from my surgery."

—*Debbie*

DEBBIE

At the time of my surgery I did not have a breast cancer diagnosis. There was a chance that the "highly suspicious mass" (that I could actually feel) was a fibroid or a cyst. In retrospect unlike my husband and parents, I was fairly confident that I didn't have cancer at all. I was sure that all our running around to doctors for tests and opinions would soon be over. My family would no longer have that worried look in their eyes, and life would get back to normal. I just knew that there was something inside me "of concern", and I wanted it out!

My personal worries at the time were not as heavy as they could have been. I was mainly concerned about how soon they could perform the surgery (my lumpectomy) and how long the recovery would be. I was totally unprepared for the path my life would take, as I was woke up from my surgery.

DONNA

My friend, and co-author Cindy, who I met at the support group, came over to my house with her mom the night before my surgery. My mom and I asked a million and one questions and they patiently answered all of them. This put our minds at ease knowing that we had a better understanding of what to expect. My parents came down from Orlando to stay with me and support me through this ordeal. Cindy also told me what to bring with me to the hospital to make the stay more comfortable. This trip wasn't going to be like a week at the Ritz.

I was so busy with my job right up to the day before my surgery. I was trying to delegate my jobs out to other employees to work on while I took some "time off". I wasn't sure how long it would be before I could return to work. Being busy up to the last hour was a blessing in disguise. I didn't have much down time to dwell on what I was up against. Before I knew it, I was being rolled off to the operating room.

TAMARA

I needed space and understanding. I needed everyone to know that I would be fundamentally different—not myself—and to be OK with that. There is a big fear that you will never be the same or normal again, and you worry about how everyone in your life will deal with that. Physically I needed help with daily tasks around the house. I also had to realize for a time that I could not do everything I was doing before. Emotionally I needed my husband to understand that I was losing everything about me that made me feel sexy. My hair, my breast, my body. Being newly married, that was terrifying!

JACKIE

Preparing for my mastectomy didn't entail any special plan. It wasn't a celebrated time or a mourned one. I didn't have a ceremony or pay tribute to my breasts. It was just something that had to be done. It was performed as soon I could possibly have it scheduled after learning that I had breast cancer. I was in no condition to "sleep on it", let alone drag it out. All I could think about was my husband and my three children and not being ready to die. The best way I can describe preparing for my mastectomy is that it was a "farewell to cancer" and that was it!

CINDY

About a week before my surgery, I started melting down. I had anxiety, I cried all the time. I was afraid. I didn't know how I would face the upcoming surgery. Even though I had the wisdom and information from my cancer sisters, I still didn't feel prepared for the surgery.

Here I was: single, never married, no children and no boyfriend. I couldn't even fathom how I would get through the next few months let alone ever find a man who would someday be interested in me sexually. My therapist suggested a healing circle to help prepare me for the surgery. She told me to invite six women who I felt close with to the circle. Each woman would provide strength and positive energy from different areas of my life. The healing circle was everything I needed it to be—deeply spiritual, emotional and comforting. It put me in the right emotional place before surgery.

After the healing circle, my circle of six threw me a Boob Voyage party complete with t-shirts that read "Boob Voyage 2006—Support the Cause."

The day of my surgery I went to the ocean to watch the sunrise. I had a private farewell with my body. I've never been madly in love with my body but I actually really liked by breasts. I took myself to the beach at sunrise to thank my body for the amazing years of health and strength. For me, making time to "thank" my body was important.

My surgery was scheduled for 11:30 am on Thursday April 6, 2006. I had to get to the hospital around 7 am for the sentinel node biopsy. I had heard tons of different things about the shots they give you for the sentinel node biopsy. I heard that it ranged from excruciating to not so bad on the pain-o-meter. For me, the pain was minimal, like a bee sting. I remember thanking the doctor for making it so tolerable. She told me she had never been thanked before.

As it often happens, my surgeon was running late so I don't think the surgery started until after 3:30 pm. I remember being told I could take a Xanax in the morning, but because of the delay, I think they started giving me anti-anxiety medicine through my IV. I remember my plastic surgeon stopping by to draw on my breasts with a purple marker. The last thing I remember was having my friends and family walk along side my bed as the nurses wheeled me down to surgery.

Next thing I knew, the surgery was over. I was being wheeled from recovery into my room. I am told I talked to my family and friends but I have no idea what we actually said. Jackie swears I was singing. It's possible—I tend to be at my funniest when I'm anxious or apparently drugged.

Once the anesthesia fog lifted, I noticed I was bandaged and had two drains on each side. The nurses gave me a morphine drip to continually provide pain relief. While on a constant drip, I had a button I could push to self medicate if the pain became intolerable. I think I only pumped the morphine two times on the second day.

From the moment I returned home, I remember trying to "walk the wall". This was advice, given to me by other Cancer Sisters, was to stand against a wall or door frame and start walking up the wall with my fingers to stretch out my arms and shoulders after surgery to prevent frozen shoulder. My pain level was probably the worst the second and third days I was home from the hospital. I didn't like taking the narcotic pain medicine so I used Tylenol and Advil to help with discomfort.

It took awhile to get used to not sleeping on my side. I bought a "study pillow" to help keep me propped up. It was months before I could lie on my side and I find that today I still tend to sleep on my back.

I went back to work three weeks after surgery but more importantly started driving about two and a half weeks after surgery once I proved to my family that I could handle turning the wheel of the car in a supermarket parking lot. To ease seatbelt discomfort I purchased a lambskin cover which helped considerably. It took a good few months until I could close my car trunk easily.

With surgery complete, healing underway and reconstruction starting, the only thing I now faced was finalizing my treatment plan based on my pathology reports.

HELPFUL TIPS FOR YOUR HOSPITAL VISIT

Make sure there is someone with you to write down all the medications you will be given.

When receiving medicine be sure you are told what it is and what it is for. When in doubt, ask a doctor.

Limit visitors. This is a very exhausting and overwhelming surgery, both physically and emotionally.

Bringing your own pillow and an "eye mask" for sleeping, can be a source of comfort.

Remind all nurses and technicians not to take your vital statistics on your affected arm. If both breasts were impacted, an ankle cuff can be used to take your blood pressure.

Bring a button down shirt for when you leave (and for future doctor visits), to ease the discomfort of having to raise your arms.

If possible try to arrange to have a private room.

Small pillows will provide comfort under your arms while you are in bed.

RECONSTRUCTION

"When my treatments were over, I wanted to look good again even if my chest lacked sensation. I knew that my new breasts would merely be a window dressing. My windows, however, would be dressed as fabulously as those in front of Macy's at Christmas."

—Gina

GINA

My plastic surgeon said to me "the reason we do reconstruction is to help women feel whole again." To me, that sums it up. I chose to have reconstructive surgery because I couldn't imagine myself without breasts. In Florida where I live, bathing suit season is year round. I did feel somewhat guilty about my attachment to my figure. After all, I was supposed to have some magical new wisdom that comes with a cancer diagnosis. Some amazing shift in priorities should have occurred. How could I be so tied to my physical appearance? Surely, some superficial, cultural expectations would not matter to me, but they did matter. When my treatments were over, I wanted to look good again even if my chest lacked sensation. I knew that my new breasts would merely be a window dressing. My windows, however, would be dressed as fabulously as those in front of Macy's at Christmas.

I decided to begin the reconstructive procedure at the time of my mastectomy. For me, the process involved the use of tissue expanders which, when filled, would create a space for implants. This procedure is sometimes referred to as TEI (tissue expander/implant). At the time of my mastectomy, temporary tissue expanders were placed under the pectoral muscle. A tissue substitute called Alloderm was also used to help create the pockets.

Over the course of about six weeks they were slowly filled to allow the skin and surrounding tissue to stretch. This is done through a port in the tissue expander. The doctor uses a little device resembling a stud finder to locate the port. He then uses a large hypodermic needle to inject saline into the port. I remember feeling tightness throughout my chest and between my shoulder blades for a day or two after each expansion. I was so uncomfortable I was irritable. Approximately 3 months after my chemotherapy and radiation was over the expanders were removed and saline implants took their place in a second surgery. As breast cancer survivors, we can choose saline or silicone implants. There are subtle differences between the two which should be discussed with a surgeon.

Unfortunately, my radiated side was slow to heal, which lead to complications. Several more surgeries were required. At times it seemed like I was running a marathon and the finish line kept getting moved! It was my plastic surgeon and his nurse Jackie that kept me going, assuring me that eventually I would make it across. The end result was worth it and I am rocking a 36C bra today.

Nipples? Yes, please. Some women forgo, for cosmetic reasons, getting new nipples. Some just get tattoos and some do both. I chose to have this surgery as well, using skin from the local area. I carefully chose the size and shape, happy to have some control. Although they don't act like nipples, sometimes when I walk into a cold room, I could swear they are getting hard. I call this the phantom nipple sensation. Imaginary or not, I'll take it.

DONNA

I chose to have a double mastectomy with immediate reconstruction. My doctor and I chose the "skin sparring" method of reconstruction. My plastic surgeon saved all my existing skin on both breast except for a small portion of skin by the tumor site and the nipples. I had a lot of skin left over from my "full DD's". I remember he had the excess skin tapped-up on the lower portion of my breast. He said the skin will shrink back to normal in a few weeks, and it did! It was amazing, I guess it's like a pregnant woman's belly shrinking back to normal after delivery, or so they hope. I never had children, so this phenomenon was new to me.

By keeping most of my skin, this helped my surgeon get in a nice size implant into my chest cavity at time of surgery. I did not have tissue expanders put in because I went with the Becker Implant. This is an implant that consists of fifty percent saline and fifty percent silicone. This implant was appealing to me because I would not need to have a second surgery to replace tissue expanders with a final implant. My implants are adjustable in size. This is a wonderful thing, I could watch them be filled with saline and decide how big I wanted to be. I had enough skin for stretching, so as my implants were expanded it did not hurt.

My surgeon used a product called "AlloDerm" in the reconstruction process. AlloDerm is cadaver skin. Due to the fact that all breast tissue was removed, the implants were placed under the chest muscle. The chest muscle only covers a portion of your breast. AlloDerm is used on the lower portion of the breast and is stitched to the pectoral muscle to give support and coverage. Not quite as nice as the first pair God gave me, but I'm grateful to have the "girls".

What helped me most during the recovery of my double mastectomy was my Mom! My mom came to stay with me for two weeks after the surgery. I only needed her to stay for one week, but like my moms do, she insisted on two. My mom took great care of me; she cooked, cleaned, shopped, emptied my drains, took care of my cats and was my personal chauffer. It sure was wonderful! If I could only get her to do that all year round!

Sleeping was hard and so was getting in a comfortable position in bed. For several weeks after surgery, I could only sleep on my back. My friend Cindy passed on arm pillows to me which were a Godsend. The small rectangular shaped pillows would go underneath each arm and made sleeping in a propped up position more comfortable.

Another big portion of my recovery was PILLS, ah, welcome to the world of pills. I found out the hard way that there is a pill for everything; pain, nausea, insomnia, constipation, neuropathy, infections, hives, burns and the list goes on. If there is a pill for it, I have tried it. Did you know that there are pills to help with the side effects of other pills?

JACKIE

Having breasts has a lot to do with how I feel as a woman. It is part of what makes me feel feminine and sexy. I also have teenagers. By nature, teenagers are very concerned about appearances.

The best way I can explain how I was feeling was when one of my daughter's friends asked her, "How does your mom have boobs? I thought she had breast cancer." Almost instinctively when people hear you have had a mastectomy they look at your chest.

The choice wasn't whether or not to do reconstruction, just what type of reconstructive surgery I would have

Regardless of the type of reconstructive surgery you have it is important to keep in mind is that it is not "enhancement surgery". They are removing all of your breast tissue and you will lose all feeling in your breasts, a sensation that takes a while to get adjusted to experiencing. I know I made the right choice for me. It has helped me and my family move forward and heal.

CINDY

I chose reconstruction at the time of my surgery. When I came out of surgery I actually was a small B cup down from my original 36Ds. I remember being surprised that they still kind of looked like breasts. Sure there was no nipple and there were stitches and drains, but I felt relieved when I saw they there were indeed small looking breasts.

I was honestly never repulsed or disgusted by my new breasts. I knew they were "under construction" and this roadwork was necessary to remove the cancer and hopefully prevent it from ever returning.

TAMARA

Having reconstructive surgery for me was not a difficult decision. I was only 31 years old and newly married. My husband and I really enjoy outdoor and water activities. I wanted to continue to be able to wear a bathing suit confidently. For me, I knew having breasts was important. A mastectomy was called for on my left breast because there were two separate lumps in different quadrants. So, trusting modern medicine and hoping for the best, I decided to have a bilateral mastectomy.

Something important that I learned was not to look at reconstruction pictures on the internet before talking to your surgeon. The pictures I found online were terrifying. Especially since there are so many different kinds of reconstruction surgeries and each one has a unique set of attributes. My plastic surgeon had many realistic pictures; however, he only showed me one of someone with similar attributes to me. He said he did not want to overwhelm me and wanted me to have a realistic picture of what the outcome of my surgery could look like.

Looking back, it was the best decision for me. I was very pleasantly surprised with my results. In fact, I was so confident on a recent vacation with my husband that I went topless on the beach in Jamaica.

HELPFUL TIPS FOR RECOVERY
FROM A LUMPECTOMY OR MASTECTOMY
SUPPORTING YOUR PHYICAL WELL-BEING:

Healthy eating
Vitamin supplements
Massages
Exercise and light stretching
Physical Therapy
Make arrangements for help with household chores, child care and pet care
Small rectangular arm pillows for sleeping

SUPPORTING YOUR EMOTIONAL WELL-BEING:

Embrace the love and support from family and friends
Remind yourself that others, even strangers are wishing good thoughts for you
Keep get well cards and letters around you
Do things that comfort you and keep your mind occupied

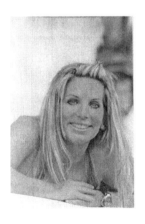
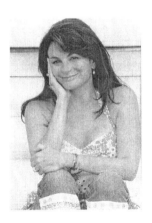

As we shared our emotional struggles regarding surgery we tried to answer some of the unknowns for you. We hope to have empowered you by reflecting on the various steps and concerns we faced during this part of our journey.

THE MEDICAL TEAM:

MEDICAL ONCOLOGIST

Charles L. Vogel, MD

Dr. Charles Vogel was trained at Princeton University and Yale Medical School. He did his Internship and Residency at Grady Memorial Hospital in association with Emory University. Thereafter for four years, he was at the Solid Tumor Branch of the National Cancer Institute in Bethesda, Maryland. For four years he was loaned by the U.S. Government to the Uganda Government to establish a Cancer Center in Uganda, East Africa where he studied primarily liver cancer, hepatoma, and Kaposi's sarcoma, which subsequently became the Caner associated with AIDS some 10 years later. In 1973, he became an Associate Professor at Emory University and started the first Oncology Ward at Grady Memorial Hospital. After two years there, he was asked by Dr. C. Gordon Zubrod to head a Division of Breast Cancer at the University of Miami's new comprehensive Cancer Center. Since 1986, he has organized clinical research programs for a number of nonprofit research entities. He is currently the Scientific Advisor for the Cancer Research Network in Boca Raton, Florida and also the Scientific Advisor for Breast Cancer Research for Aptium Oncology located at the Lynn Regional Cancer Institute West in Boca Raton.

THE ROLE OF AN ONCOLOGIST IN BREAST CANCER TREATMENT

There are different forms of oncologists including medical, surgical, and radiation oncologists. The Medical Oncologist, after surgery usually is the "Captain of the team." Breast cancer treatment is a team approach that includes those other oncologic specialties as well as pathology, social work, psychiatry, reconstructive surgery, and many other subspecialists. The Medical Oncologist orchestrates all of the drug treatments that are used to help manage breast cancer patients. These include antihormal therapy, strong drugs which are commonly called chemotherapy and the newer targeted therapies. Many Oncologists also participate in a broad range of clinical research programs in order to provide cutting edge treatments to their patients. Many of the newer more exciting drugs are available only in an investigational setting and Oncologists who do not participate in clinical research, often do not have access to these exciting and potentially paradigm changing treatments.

THOUGHTS ON THE FUTURE OF BREAST CANCER TREATMENT

I would like to see chemotherapy as we currently define it, disappear from our armamentarium and be replaces by drugs that are less indiscriminate in terms of their effect on normal cells of the body. Antihormonal therapy tends to be kinder, gentler therapy, and targeted therapies, while having unique toxicities of their own, stand a better chance of being more specific and less indiscriminate in their toxicity patterns. I am also hoping that someday there will be a blood test that will be reliable in predicting early breast cancer, but such a test has been elusive in coming.

I have been encouraged by the reduced role of surgery in accomplishing its goal with less mutilating procedures.

GREATEST ACHIEVEMENTS TO DATE FOR YOUNG WOMEN WITH A BREAST CANCER DIAGNOSIS

Genetic testing and counseling has been important in helping to identify the highest risk women, who more commonly occur in the younger age groups. By identifying such women even before breast cancer develops, allows for the use of preventative therapies that can markedly reduces the risk of their developing this dread disease. The use of earlier and stronger forms of chemotherapy and antihormonal therapy have also played a major role in leading to a decrease in mortality from breast cancer in younger women, while the use of less mutilating surgery has lead to a better cosmetic result in such women. Even those who must have a mastectomy because of the types of cancer they have, can be made more "whole" again through the use of reconstructive techniques.

A PERSONAL NOTE FROM THE DOCTOR:

I chose this field of medicine because Oncology is so rapidly changing and advances occur yearly if not in some cases even more frequently. We have so many tools in our armamentarium to help breast cancer patients that is why this is a very rewarding field. Most of my patients are cured even through many have to go through the rigors of surgery, radiation, and chemotherapy to achieve that goal. Even for the percent of women who have not been cured and have metastatic disease, we have so many different treatments that we can prolong and optimize their life, often with minimal symptoms and minimal hospitalizations, often for years. I have so many rewarding experiences that they are too numerous to recount. From the standpoint of my research involvement, I will always be thankful that I was able to have the opportunity to be on the ground floor of Herceptin research and to be one of the main figures in the field of early Herceptin clinical research. My long career in breast cancer oncology has led me to be involved in the development of virtually every single breast cancer drug that is now in common place use for our patient population. Without my continuing role in cutting edge research, my role as an oncologist, would be less fruitful in my own eyes, and make me less of an asset to my patients.

ONCOLOGY NURSE

Alisha Stein, RNC, BSN, OCN

Alisha received her Bachelor's of Science Degree in Psychology with a minor in Education from the University of Florida. She subsequently went on to study nursing at Barry University, and has maintained her nursing career solely in oncology. Her background includes both inpatient and outpatient settings. She has spent the last 5 years working closely with Dr. Charles Vogel and the Cancer Research Network (www.crninc.org) specializing in breast cancer and breast cancer research. She is passionate about breast cancer care and Cancer Research Network's (CRN) mission. CRN is dedicated to improving the standard of cancer care through clinical research, education, advocacy, and community outreach. CRN's advocacy and community outreach initiatives help cancer patients and caregivers cope with the disease and assist in the management of everyday struggles they face from diagnosis through survivorship. Alisha's experience as a breast cancer nurse has enabled her to be an active voice in the community, and in oncology nursing.

THE ROLE OF THE ONCOLOGY NURSE

The oncology nurses you encounter before, during, and after your treatment will wear many hats. They are a critical link to your care, and will guide you through the many transitions involved from your initial diagnosis to, the completion of your treatment, into a world of breast cancer survivors. You and your loved ones may be overwhelmed with questions, concerns, and confusion; your oncology nurses will be there for you. They are a wealth of information, and they will keep you informed about the medications you will be receiving, as well as possible side effects. They are the problem solvers when it comes to preventing and managing side effects, and the shoulder to lean on when you need support. Please share your experiences (whether you believe them to be related to your treatment or not) with your nurses, and they will guide you.

BREAKTHROUGHS IN SUPPORTIVE CARE

One of the greatest breakthroughs in oncology nursing in addition to the advances in the prevention and management of nausea and vomiting is the use of Colony Stimulating Factors like Neulasta and Neupogen. Historically, chemotherapy induced neutropenia (a decrease in the cells that help prevent infection) has been a major dose limiting toxicity associated with treatment. Patient's treatments would be delayed until their cell counts improved and/or their chemotherapy dosages would be reduced. Studies such as the Bonadonna study (1995), have shown that patients receive the greatest benefit from their chemotherapy treatment when they receive >/= 85% of their planned chemotherapy dose.

Use of Colony Stimulating Factors has enabled oncologists and oncology nurses to maintain treatment schedules and dosages, and maximize the benefits of chemotherapy.

THE IMPORTANCE OF CLINICAL TRIALS AND THE FUTURE OF BREAST CANCER

At times it is difficult for health care providers and the public to recognize the advances made in breast cancer through research. Clinical trials are the means to hopefully one day finding a cure. We would still be performing radical mastectomies on all women diagnosed with breast cancer had clinical trials not shown us that a lumpectomy plus radiation has equal benefit. It is through clinical trials that chemotherapy options have been identified and most recently the use of targeted therapies. At one point or another we have all asked ourselves "what is taking so long to find a cure?" Only 3% of adult cancer patients participate in clinical trials. Why? There are an enumerable amount of myths associated with research. The greatest myth is the belief that one will be used as a "guinea pig." There are no guinea pigs in the clinical setting. Yes, of course preclinical studies are conducted, but this is long before studies are implemented with people. In cancer research patients will receive what is presently considered to be the best standard of therapy or the therapy being studied which is believed to be equal or superior to the present standard. The only way to answer this question is through a clinical trial. Her2 positive patients did not start receiving Herceptin in the early stage breast cancer setting until 2005 when the results of clinical trials demonstrated that adding Herceptin to chemotherapy (which was the standard) was more beneficial than chemotherapy alone.

There are many clinical trials in progress that will aid in answering many unanswered questions in breast cancer. One of the most exciting trials for HER2+ patients in the early stage breast cancer setting is the ALLTO study. Patients in this study will receive Tykerb an oral targeted therapy, or Herceptin, or the combination of the two drugs together or sequentially with Herceptin for three months followed by Tykerb.

A PERSONAL NOTE FROM THE ONCOLOGY NURSE

As you are faced with many decisions in regards with how to proceed with your breast cancer treatment explore the potential to participate in a clinical trial. You are not alone, remember the wise words the six young women shared with you in this book, and remember you are in control.

RECONSTRUCTIVE SURGERY

Andrew H. Rosenthal, MD

Dr. Rosenthal is Board Certified by the American Board of Plastic Surgery. He completed his internship in surgery at the University of Miami, before beginning an intensive six-year integrated program in Plastic Surgery at The University of Michigan Hospital. In addition to his work in Plastic Surgery, Dr. Rosenthal also completed a two-year research fellowship while at the University of Michigan where he focused on difficult problems in pediatric facial reconstruction, leading to his invention of a device to help prevent positional head deformity in children.

Dr. Rosenthal is also a published author in cosmetic, breast, face, and hand surgery. His articles have appeared in the prestigious Journal of Plastic and Reconstructive Surgery and in Plastic Surgical Forum. He holds degrees with honors from Duke University and Tulane University Medical School, where he was elected as a member of Alpha Omega Alpha, a national honor reserved for top medical school graduates.

BREAST RECONSTRUCTION USING IMPLANTS

Synthetic implants are pouches that are placed under a layer of chest muscle to create the shape of a breast. The outside of the implant is made of a solid silicone shell and it is filled with silicone gel or saline. Saline is another word for salt water. Silicone is an artificial material that feels like natural breast tissue. Most commonly, implant breast reconstruction is carried out in two stages. The first stage consists of placement of a device called a "tissue expander." An expander is a silicone-walled pouch that resembles an empty balloon with a small port in its front wall. This valve allows the surgeon to fill the implant with saline in the weeks following this initial operation. This initial surgery takes approximately one to two hours and can be performed at the time of mastectomy or afterwards ("delayed reconstruction"). During the second stage, the tissue expander is replaced with an implant.

Approximately 10 to 21 days following placement of the tissue expander, the process of tissue expansion will begin. Every one to two weeks, you will visit your plastic surgeon. During these 20- to 30-minute visits, approximately two to four ounces of saline (salt water) will be injected through the overlying skin into the port located on the front wall of the tissue expander. This is done with a fine needle.

With each visit, the tissue expander is gradually inflated. The growing tissue expander enlarges the pocket, inducing growth of the overlying skin. In essence, this tissue expander grows the skin for the new breast. The expansion process causes slight soreness or discomfort in some women while others report simply a feeling of "tightness" for several days following each expansion.

Approximately one to three months after the tissue expander has reached the correct size, you will undergo a second operation. During this surgery, the expander is removed and an implant is inserted in its place. The surgery lasts about one to two hours and you can usually go home the day of surgery.

NATURAL TISSUE RECONSTRUCTION

A natural tissue reconstruction procedure is when your own body tissue can be used to recreate a breast. The most common kind of natural tissue reconstruction is the TRAM, in which tissue from the abdomen is used to create the breast.

Natural tissue reconstruction can also be done using other sites:

TRAM (Transverse Rectus Abdominis Muscle) Flap Reconstruction and DIEP/SIEA flap reconstruction

This operation uses tissue from your lower abdomen to make a new breast. It can either be done with the tissue remaining connected and tunneled under your abdominal muscle and skin ("pedicled" TRAM) or with the tissue disconnected from the abdomen and reattached on the chest ("free" or microsurgical TRAM). Newer procedures which spare the abdominal muscle are also available now (DIEP or SIEA flap).

NIPPLE RECONSTRUCTION

Nipple and areola (the dark circle around the nipple) reconstruction is completely optional. Some women want only the shape of the breast to fill a bra, and decide they don't need a nipple. Another option is to apply removable nipples that stick on with adhesive. These rubbery tips are shaped like a semi-erect nipple and the color and texture are quite lifelike.

NIPPLE RECONSTRUCTION PROCEDURE

If you choose to surgically reconstruct the nipple, there are several options. One common option is to use the skin of your reconstructed breast. The surgeon can take a small flap of skin from the breast, and "cone" it into a new nipple. Because the nerves aren't connected in the reconstructed breast, most women do not feel much pain with this surgery.

Options to reconstruct the areola involve taking skin from a different part of the body and sewing it to the new nipple on the reconstructed breast. The surgeon can take an circle of skin from the outer edge of your mastectomy scar or from the edge of the TRAM donor scar on your abdomen (if you have this kind of breast reconstruction). The advantage of using this skin is that you won't have any new scars. The surgeon can also take skin from the inside of your thigh or from just below your hip bone. You may be sore for up to two weeks at the place from which the skin was taken. However, most women have very little discomfort at the site of the reconstructed nipple. Another option is to reconstruct the nipple as described above and have the skin around it tattooed to a darker color to make an areola.

In all procedures, you will not have much or any feeling in the new nipple when it is touched. These surgeries can be done on an outpatient basis in less than two hours, with local or general anesthesia.

After you have healed, you can have the new nipple and areola tattooed to match the color of your other nipple. Often it takes two or three sessions to color the whole area evenly.

WHEN IS NIPPLE RECONSTRUCTION PERFORMED?

Most plastic surgeons do not schedule nipple reconstruction until there has been time for the swelling from the previous surgery to go down and for the breast to "settle." This allows the surgeon to place the nipple so that it matches the position of the nipple on the other breast.

INFORMATION FOR CANCER PATIENTS TO CONSIDER:

THE EFFECTS OF CHEMOTHERAPY AND RADIATION ON BREAST RECONSTRUCTION

Radiation can negatively impact breast reconstruction both tissue expanders/ implants and autogenous (produced using tissue from your own body). Autogenous tissue usually fares better however. The most common complication from radiation with tissue expanders and implants is capsular contracture—that is the scar capsule surrounding the implant becomes hard and may not look right and may even be painful. Irradiated tissues are also more susceptible to infection and may not heal properly. If you know you are going to need radiation, it is sometimes better to wait for reconstruction ("delayed reconstruction"). This is especially true if you are considering an autogenous reconstruction because that way this tissue from another part of the body won't have been irradiated and bringing in this healthy tissue can actually help the area heal.

Chemotherapy usually does not affect the quality of a breast reconstruction. However, it can make you more susceptible to infections related to your reconstruction.

THE ROLE OF EMOTIONS

As a plastic & reconstructive surgeon, I deal with a portion of the cancer treatment that is often the most satisfying to patients—making them feel whole again. Certainly breast cancer is an emotional rollercoaster with many unexpected twists and turns. The reconstructive process can add to the stress because it is a complicated process by itself. However, the final result is tangible things which can often help patients heal on a different level.

HOW TO CHOOSE A RECONSTRUCTIVE SURGEON

Make sure your plastic surgeon is certified or eligible for certification by the American Board of Plastic and Reconstructive Surgery.

As him or her how many surgeries of this type s/he does. This doesn't have to be the ONLY thing they do, but they should do it more than a few times a year.

As to speak to other patients who have been through the type of reconstruction you are choosing or those you are choosing between. I find this much more helpful than photos. Many patients ask for photos, but anatomy is very individualized and it does not mean you will look like that. Remember your surgeon is probably only going to choose his or her best results to show you. And you don't want to look at photos of breast AUGMENTATIONS. Augmentations and reconstructions are very, very different.

Also ask what types of breast reconstruction s/he does. Even if the surgeon doesn't offer, ask about the other types and why they weren't discussed. If s/he is discussing only one type is may be because that is the only type s/he knows or does.

Ask for educational materials and resources. It is very difficult to remember everything your doctor said (studies say people only retain about 30%). And ask for online resources s/he trusts—the internet is rife with misinformation. Also bring someone with you (family member or friend) who can make notes or at least listen with you. Don't be afraid to call back or ask for an email contact to ask more questions.

Choose your reconstructive surgeon carefully—remember this is going to be a long relationship.

Lastly, don't be afraid to NOT have reconstruction or to delay reconstruction. Sometimes it is just too much to take in and too many decisions to make in the whirlwind of a diagnosis of cancer. It's ok to hold off on reconstruction Just make sure you understand the pluses and minuses of doing so.

GREATEST ACHIEVEMENTS TO DATE FOR YOUNG WOMEN WITH A BREAST CANCER DIAGNOSIS

Recent research has shown that, regardless of age, most women identify their breasts as their most important aesthetic center and the feature which most prominently makes them identify with being a woman and being attractive. The biggest thing I can share with young women diagnosed with breast cancer is that there is life after breast cancer. Just about everybody can get reconstruction. There are many different methods and you need to do your homework and find out what is right for you—now and for the long term. Breast reconstruction after cancer can give you the confidence to face the future and to not feel like something was "taken" from you.

A PERSONAL NOTE FROM THE DOCTOR

My mother was also diagnosed with breast cancer. I enjoy the ability to interact with women undergoing the reconstructive process and in taking a part in making them "whole" again. In fact, I often am continuing to work putting the finishing touches on long after many of the rest of the cancer team is done. I do perform significant amounts of cosmetic surgery of the breast as well as the rest of the body because that type of experience enhances my ability to "think outside the box" in solving difficult reconstructive breast problems and coming up with new solutions to old problems.

I enjoy breast cancer reconstruction because I find the patients to be very grateful, because I find the surgeries challenging yet satisfying, and because it is true plastic surgery—making something out of nothing.

CHAPTER FOUR

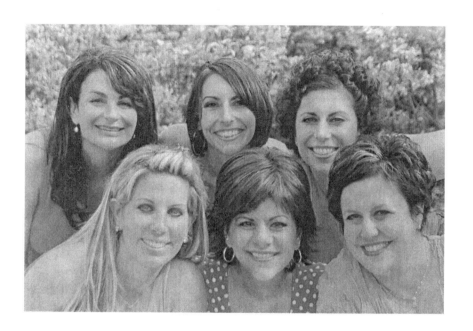

TREATMENT:
TRUE WARRIORS

"It has taken some time, and the scar from my port is barely visible, but once in a while I will catch a glimpse of it and I actually feel proud. I feel a sense of accomplishment. It is my badge of bravery and a subtle reminder to me that I can accomplish just about anything, even if it seems impossible."

—Debbie

This section of the book deals with the "nuts and bolts" of your breast cancer journey. It is also a section to which we have so much to offer given the gift of hindsight. There is advice we wish we had been given and the experiences to back it up. We openly discuss the port, chemotherapy, radiation, hormonal therapy and more. Although everyone's experience will vary, remember you are not alone because there are also many similarities among women's struggles.

THE PORT

JACKIE

As my breast cancer diagnosis sank in and I realized that chemotherapy was my best option for getting rid of any possible cancer left in my body, I wanted to start getting treatment immediately. My doctor assured me that we were proceeding in a timely manner, but that I needed to have a port put in first. His next words were, "It's a very minor surgery."

I had just had a double mastectomy (I still wasn't over the shock from that), I finally had the drains removed from my chest, I was beginning to get mobility back in my arms and all I could hear was him saying was that I would need to have another surgery! I really didn't understand what a port was; I was too overwhelmed to ask questions, I was afraid and I didn't want it. I told my doctor to start mixing my drugs because I would be there tomorrow morning for my treatment.

It is not mandatory to have a port. So, I showed up, as promised, and proceeded to have four chemotherapy treatments without a port. As they began my fifth treatment, the chemotherapy drugs began to burn through my veins. Immediately, the drugs began spreading through my body, releasing the toxins. When that happens, the procedure is to try to move to another vein in a higher location. By this time, I was in extreme distress and unable to continue with my chemotherapy.

The next day I made an appointment to have a port put in. It was a small device placed just under the skin in my arm. It was inserted with a local anesthetic and was relatively painless, especially compared to the trauma of the chemotherapy burn.

The result of using my veins instead of a port was months and months of daily physical therapy that was hours long. My arm looked horrible, felt horrible and had to be wrapped at all times. It was wrapped with different kinds of bandages and a compression sleeve 23 hours a day. Some of the harm from the burn is still a chronic issue for me.

Receiving chemotherapy through a vein instead of a port does not automatically equal an experience like I had. However, looking back, it really wasn't a big deal to have the port put in, it made it very simple to receive chemotherapy and have blood drawn and it came out without difficulty.

DEBBIE

I was told by my oncologist that I would need to get a port before chemotherapy began. I remember vaguely understanding what that meant. Still, I dutifully set up the surgery appointment as I left the office.

About a week later a double port was placed on the right side of my chest just under the skin. I was put under twilight anesthesia. There was a very tiny scar (which I still have today) but other than that it was not noticeable. It was only uncomfortable in the sense that I knew it was there. Numerous blood draws, too many to count, and the chemotherapy medications were either taken out or put into my body via the port. Although I knew this little plastic device was playing a major role in my fight against cancer, I couldn't help myself from resenting it. For me, it represented cancer in every way, shape and form.

The day my port was removed was, needless to say, a great day! I felt I was finally given the opportunity to move on. It has taken some time, and the scar from my port is barely visible, but once in a while I will catch a glimpse of it and I actually feel proud. I feel a sense of accomplishment. It is my badge of bravery and a subtle reminder to me that I can accomplish just about anything, even if it seems impossible.

TAMARA

I chose to have a port placed at my initial surgery, my mastectomy. I was aware that I would need chemotherapy for a full year. Some of the chemotherapy drugs can destroy your veins and cause sloughing of the skin if it gets out of the vein. I didn't want to worry each time whether or not the nurse was going to be able to find a vein.

I had my port inserted under the skin on my chest. I was comfortable with it there because it was out of the way for the most part. It was very visible though as was the tube that was connected to my vein. To me, it looked a little odd, like I had an angry vein. It really didn't bother me until my chemotherapy was over. I had to leave the port in for anther year to receive my Herceptin treatments every three weeks. It upset me because I felt I was finally getting back to normal. My hair was growing in and I had finished all my reconstruction surgeries. Still, my port was always drawing attention.

The port removal day was very significant for me. I didn't think the removal of it would matter as much as it did. I had been living with it for a year. I was amazed at how much better I felt when it was gone. It was the last external evidence of my battle with cancer. Outwardly I was normal again. I was no longer a cancer patient!

GINA

The chemotherapy process begins with a minor surgical procedure to put in a port a catheter. It is a special valve placed under the skin that has a direct line into a main artery. It is the safest way to deliver the medicine and spare the veins. It stays in place during the entire course of treatment.

At the time, it was the norm to have it in your chest. An advocate suggested I consider getting it in my arm beside my bicep, I liked the idea. My surgeon did not. I had said I didn't want the visible scar on my chest because I like to wear jewelry, he said wear bigger jewelry. Ignoring his insensitive remark and refusing the old standard, I persisted. Eventually, he acquiesced and told me where I could get the arm port. The process only took a few hours.

This was a hard step, because when I was diagnosed I didn't feel sick, certainly didn't think of myself as sick. As a matter of fact, I thought I was in the best shape of my life. But when they put in the port, suddenly I felt like a cancer patient, the disease was undeniable. The device seems like something out of a science fiction novel. A weird alien like bump that separates you from all the healthy humans.

It was the beginning of my fight. Now that my port had been removed, it seems fitting that I have a scar over my bicep, the modern day symbol of strength. When I see it, I feel stronger. Today, just a short time after I bucked the system, many women choose to get an arm port.

CINDY

A couple of weeks prior to chemotherapy I had my arm port put in via out-patient surgery. I elected to have an arm port put in versus having a chest port or no port at all. This would make it easer to administer the chemotherapy and less likely that I would have vein damage. I chose an arm port over a chest port. I figured an arm scar would be less visible than a chest scar—especially for those daring/baring tops I would certainly soon be wearing! The port was a little uncomfortable at first—bruised and swollen—but I am absolutely happy with decision to place it in my arm! About three weeks after my last chemotherapy session they removed the port—another out-patient procedure.

DONNA

I was told that because of the harshness of the chemotherapy drugs on your veins that I would need to have a port temporarily implanted to receive treatments. Some of the girls in the support group had their ports put in their upper chest and some had them put in their arm by their bi-cep. I chose to put my port in my arm because I felt like I already had enough scars on my chest, why add another one to it? It left a scar about one inch long on the inside of my arm. To me, this area is less obvious than the chest. Some girls complained about the chest port getting in the way of their bra strap or seat belt as well.

I think that the port looks ugly, whether it is in the arm or chest. It looks like an alien is living under the skin. Either way, it can be painful when it is accidentally hit. The port is a small round metal device that is placed under the skin in an out-patient procedure. I was not given anesthesia, but really wished that I had been for the procedure. I found myself very stressed-out during the surgery. My whole body would start to shiver from the stress, not the cold. There is a thin tube attached to the port that is inserted into a vein and goes up the arm and terminates by your heart.

I dreaded getting my chemotherapy treatments because I started to associate the port with pain. It would hurt me when they put the needle in the port and when they took it out. I didn't want anyone messing with my port. After I finished all of my treatments, I had the port removed. Again, with nothing to calm my nerves, I couldn't bear to watch the doctor while he removed the alien from under my skin. The doctor let me keep the port as a souvenir! I now wear it as a badge of honor. I made it into a piece of jewelry. It sure makes for a good conversation starter!

CHEMOTHERAPY

"When I think about my chemotherapy experience, it's kind of bittersweet. The difficult part, of course, was the actual treatment. Yet the end result, knowing I fought cancer with all my might, that's something I'll never have to regret."

—*Jackie*

DEBBIE

As I think about what I could say with regard to chemotherapy I am assaulted with a barrage of sights, sounds and smells. I remember that, as my husband would open the door of the CTU (Chemotherapy Treatment Unit), I would be hit with its odor making the first step inside the most difficult. I learned a "new language" as the names of each drug was called and then double checked before being administered. The sea of nurses was, visible in all areas of the room, suited up and protected with gloves and masks. I will never forget the bright orange labels drawing attention to the poisonous and toxic medicine in the many syringes and bags of intravenous medications. I can still hear the beeping of the IV machines, calling out to be supplied with another dose. In some ways I can still taste the metallic flavor and smell of the drug Heprin that was used to flush out my port before each treatment began. I also recall being highly conscious of the odor from the drugs that permeated my skin for days after each treatment. The taste of the seemingly gallons of water I drank to flush out my body still lingers from time to time. In addition, the aroma of the sandwiches has stuck with me—the smell from the lunch cart would waft through the air as food was passed out for patients and their caregiver. And, as if it were background music to my play, the low hum of televisions or people talking and the gentle voices of the art therapy volunteers as they spread good will to people trying desperately to pass the time—I remember these sounds.

There were also some things that I remember as being helpful. A nurse once shared with me that if I held my nose when they administer the Heprin, I wouldn't experience the metallic taste. It worked. Drinking lots of water helped to flush out toxins. Also, taking all of the prescribed anti-nausea medications helped me to cope with many of the side-effects. I always kept in mind that I had a suppressed immune system such that I avoided places with a high risk of germs. This act helped me to be strong enough to receive all of my treatments on time. Whenever it was possible, I had my "pre-chemotherapy" blood work done the day before my scheduled treatment. I was able to alleviate the worry that I would show up and be sent home the following day without receiving my chemotherapy. I also keep a notebook where I placed copies of all blood tests, chemotherapy drug orders and other papers that contained information about me and/or my health. Being able to access these papers so easily helped me on several occasions.

Eating simply, mainly healthy foods, helped to quell the upset and shock my body was going through as the medications did their job.

There are some other memories from my chemotherapy experience that I will treasure forever. It was a highlight of my days to read the cards that were sent by family and friends. I loved to listen to the messages on my answering machine. They helped me to stay connected to the world when I didn't have the strength carry on a conversation, let alone visit with anyone. I look lovingly at my wonderful children who were so sweet to each other and snuggled with me as often as possible.

Most of all, I remember lying in my chair, with my soft pink blanket, terry cloth warm-up suit and bandana, trying my best to sleep away the hours until the treatment was over. I was so thankful that every time I opened my eyes, I saw my husband. He would sit, ever so patiently, in a chair that could be described as anything but comfortable, with a stack of magazines and newspapers. It would take but a second for him to catch my eye and send me a look that everything was going as planned and that I was going to be fine. We were going to be fine. Our family was going to be fine. It is a picture I will remember forever.

TAMARA

The best adjective that I can think of to describe chemotherapy is *rough*. My first treatment hit me hard. It was very strange to go into the chemotherapy room and get all these drugs intravenously. I could feel it go through my body and also taste some of the drugs. My vision got blurry, my head hurt and my urine smelled funny. Then, four hours later, the nausea and heartburn kicked in. It felt as though I had downed a glass of gasoline. The doctors provide a lot of drugs and steroids for the nausea. They made my heartburn worse, and I was still very nauseous. I never vomited but was wiped out and unable to get out of bed for five full days.

The first treatment also made my surgery site (where the expanders were) hurt again—just like it did about three days post surgery. I felt like I had been beaten with a bat! I had my treatments on Monday, which wiped me out for five days. By Saturday, I could get up and go to work as a vet. I just had to go slowly and take naps in between patients. My treatments were two weeks apart so on my "good" week, I would run around trying to get everything ready for my chemotherapy week. Each treatment was a little different. Some weren't so bad, others were worse. At the end of the first four treatments, I was very weak and didn't care about much of anything.

For the last four of my eight treatments, the medicines changed. My first chemotherapy with the new drug combination was great: nothing happened. I was just a little achy, and I was so relieved. My following treatment was supposed to be one week later, but my white blood cell count was low so my therapy got pushed back a week. The following week, my count was still low, so the doctor gave me a shot called Neulasta to boost up my white blood cells.

Three days later, I was at work and I started to ache all over and my fingers and toes went numb. I started hobbling around like a 90 year old woman. For five straight days I couldn't sleep because even lying down was very uncomfortable and painful. I continued to go to work, to try to keep my mind off of the pain. A few days later, I called my doctor to ask if it was supposed to be this painful. She decided on the spot to stop my treatments. Many people have adverse reactions to the drug I was receiving or are unable to tolerate it.

After that I continued with only Herceptin treatments every three weeks for a year and the feeling in my fingers and toes returned.

DONNA

My first chemotherapy treatment was the hardest for me emotionally. The hard part was I did not know what to expect or how my body would react to the vast array of chemicals. I will never forget my first treatment; it will be etched in my memory for life. My girlfriend and five women from my support group all attended that chemotherapy session. I had a full cheerleading team! As I sat in the chemotherapy chair for an hour before they actually hooked me up to the IV fluids, I began to get anxious and stressed. The girls did a great job keeping me distracted. Once the treatment actually began, the nurse informed me she would be administering the chemotherapy drugs at a slower rate in the beginning. This was to keep an eye out for any immediate adverse reactions. It is a strange concept to voluntarily sit in a chair and let a nurse put a needle in your arm and administer poison into your veins! The experience reminded me of the electric chair. My girlfriends were the witness's waiting for the moment of execution. I would ask myself, "Why was this happening to me? I didn't commit any crime". It really meant the world to me to have the girls from the support group that I had just recently met come out and support me. They are the best!

I had a total of seven chemotherapy treatments. I received chemotherapy every two weeks, but I had to skip one week because my blood counts were too low. The chemotherapy drugs actually attack red and white blood cells and lower your immune system. The following day after my treatments I would get a Nuelasta shot in my arm to boost up my blood counts. It felt like a nasty bee sting. I have a very low threshold for pain, probably equivalent to that of a two year old. It was distressing to have to submit myself to pain and needles week after week. Sadly, this becomes a common routine for most breast cancer patients. Exactly two days after my first three treatments I would have what I call "Bed Day". Although it sounds exciting to be able to stay in bed all day, it actually felt like a form of torture for me. I couldn't do anything, I felt really out of sorts and I had a hard time focusing even to watch T.V. I would sleep for a few hours, and toss and turn for a few hours. I would constantly be looking at the clock in the middle of the night, waiting for a decent hour so I could get out of bed and get on with the next day. I grew to dread "Bed Day".

There were also horrible moments of nausea that I endured. I guess that's what morning sickness might feel like. To combat some of the nausea, I was given anti-nausea drugs, which helped, I never actually threw up. Because I would feel yucky for a few days after treatment, I planned my treatments on Thursdays so that I would be sick over the weekend and not have to miss work. I usually felt good for ten days out of the two week cycle. Then, once your feeling good again, Zap, they hit you with another treatment.

I tried to go about my business as usual and did almost everything that I used to do before I had breast cancer. Sometimes I would almost forget that I had cancer, until I scratched my bald head! When my fourth chemotherapy treatment ended, I felt as if I had had enough. The side effects are cumulative and you just start to get worn out towards the end. As round five began, I was given different chemotherapy drugs. Three days after receiving the new drug, Taxol, I developed neuropathy in my hands and feet. The side effect that I experienced was numbness and a tingling sensation in my extremities. This would last for several months. I was immediately switched to a different comparable medicine for my remaining treatments.

GINA

As I sat down to write about this subject, I realized that it had been a little over a year since my last chemotherapy and just five months since my last Herceptin treatment. Amazingly, so much of my treatment process was already a blur. As it had after childbirth, my body had forgotten a lot of the details of the experience.

I remember commenting to one of my physicians that I couldn't remember much about the previous year. They commented that it was a good year to forget. Needing a little help, I recalled the journal a dear friend gave to me when I first became sick. As I reached into the top drawer of my bedside table to retrieve it, I was hopeful that I had written something during all those sleepless nights. Unfortunately, throughout the six months I was systematically poisoned, I wasn't that prolific, my journal contained only random thoughts. Some of which will help me convey the fog and total body experience that is chemotherapy.

In that beside table I also kept stacks of get well cards. One of them was singled out and placed with my medical information, it read; "courage is feeling the fear and doing it anyway." That is how it was for me. The fear was overwhelming at times, but it's amazing what you'll sign up for when faced with death. So, although my courage was barely tangible, I decided to get well. The chemotherapy process begins with a port a catheter, a special valve placed under the skin that has a direct line into a main artery. It is the safest way to deliver the medicine and spare the veins.

Waiting for my first chemotherapy treatment felt like waiting for the electric chair, perhaps worse. I should have checked out the chemotherapy room at my oncologist's office to quell some of the anxiety. As the time drew near, my fear escalated. In part because of the mental picture I had created of the weak, hairless, nauseous and emaciated cancer patient I would become. I had to take an anxiety pill just to walk in for my first treatment. Accompanied by my husband and a girlfriend (survivor) I made it through the door. I carried with me a bag of things that I thought I would need: a blanket, bottled water, crackers, hard candies, gossip magazines, a cell phone and my ipod. It was a lot of stuff, but the treatments would take approximately six hours! After a very long, emotional day, I went home and waited to feel sick. My vague notes revealed that I felt the worst on days 3–5 after chemotherapy. As the 12 treatments wore on, I tweaked my routine a bit. I preferred to go alone with a jamba juice smoothie, some Tums and my ipod. Sometimes I would even score points with the nurses by bringing them smoothies as well. Family and friends would chauffer me back and forth. The IV medications were delivered every three weeks. For fifteen months I showed up, often in the same hoodie, short sleeve t-shirt (for port access) and sweat pants. When it was over, I threw out all the clothes that reminded me of sitting in that chair.

People always want to know about the side affects, so at the risk of sounding whiney I will list some of mine. At times I experienced the following symptoms: nausea, body aches, night sweats, constipation, vision problems, loss of appetite, pain in feet, sensitivity to sound, difficulty with balance, nasal congestion, bloody noses, skin rash, diarrhea, head aches, pins and needles, insomnia, hair loss and chemo brain. I made it through with the love and support of my friends and family. My mother, in-laws and sister-in-law spent countless nights on our couch, tending to me and keeping things running smoothly. I also found a few other things to be very helpful; they were the Tivo, a lap top, meditation, a sound machine (ocean waves), Cheech and Chong, and an ipod. The ipod was great in the doctors' offices because I could put it on and disengage from all the misery and conversation that happens in waiting rooms.

The master bedroom became my domain. In anticipation of all the time I would be spending there, I bought luxurious sheets and new pillows. I stocked a little refrigerator with drinks so I wouldn't have to run downstairs. Carpets were cleaned and fresh flowers were always in view. Beautiful melon scented candles were lit and wonderful bath products were on hand. My husband graciously slept in another room for up to a week at a time so I didn't have to feel guilty about waking him throughout the night. Creature comforts were very important.

Throughout the treatment cycles, patients' lives revolve around their counts. These are the numbers used to analyze blood work. Shots are given to keep your counts up; they too can cause unpleasant side effects. When they are low, there is a greater risk of infection. So, during the six months of intense chemotherapy I avoided raw foods that may contain harmful bacteria and continued to eat healthy. I avoided large crowds. I did not participate in lunch duty at my son's elementary school. At Christmas I did not see many of my family members because they were or had been around someone who was sick. I did not fly on commercial airplanes either, not even to escape a hurricane! Once when my counts were up, I put on my wig and a hot outfit and went to a U2 concert. It was an exception that encouraged my emotional well being. All these precautions paid off because my chemotherapy remained on schedule and I was able to complete my treatment.

JACKIE

Chemotherapy was nothing like I expected. The only frame of reference I had to draw from was what I had seen in movies or on TV. Chemotherapy was awful and debilitating, but not like what I'm sure it would have been even five or six years ago thanks to the heightened level of awareness and the many advances made through research.

When I think about my chemotherapy experience, it's kind of bittersweet. The difficult part, of course, was the actual treatment. Yet the end result, knowing I fought cancer with all my might, that's something I'll never have to regret.

I experienced many of the same side effects as my cancer sisters. I felt full of the medicines, toxins, and poison. My husband often said he felt like if he had touched a light bulb to my head, it would have lit. As soon as I got home from my treatments, all I wanted to do was take a shower. The only foods that seemed to help me were baked potatoes, soup and ginger ale. The second day was always the worst, though; from the Neulasta shot (a medication that stimulates your blood cells). My body would become weak and sore. Even the slightest touch would be agonizing. I was overwhelmed and exhausted and slept often.

As my medications changed, so did my side effects. Some worse, some better. I was able to tolerate the medication I received towards the end of chemotherapy better than I had at the beginning. I began exercising again, which made me feel better. I was still tired and not yet back to myself, but I could see the end in sight.

Receiving chemotherapy treatments is difficult. But, as they say, I sat there and took my medicine. What other choice did I have? I wanted to live, and chemotherapy was part of the "prescription" to accomplish that.

CINDY

Once I decided to proceed with the bilateral mastectomy with reconstruction, the next step was to determine what my treatment plan would be. The Oncologist stressed that given the size of my tumor and my age, she highly recommended that I undergo chemotherapy. We would not know whether or not I needed radiation until we received the pathology from my mastectomy.

The pathology we received at my cancer diagnosis indicated that I was HER 2 negative and ER/PR negative. This means my cancer would not be responsive to common cancer drugs like Herceptin and Tamoxifen. For this reason, my Oncologist prescribed dose dense chemotherapy, which means treatments every two weeks. My treatment period would last for a total of 16 weeks. It was going to be a long summer!

The post mastectomy pathology confirmed there was no lymph node involvement. This meant that I would not have to add radiation to my treatment plan.

I decided to have chemotherapy on Thursdays since I'd heard that most of the side effects occur one to three days later. This way I could continue to work during the week.

I started chemotherapy at the end of April, 2006.

I was very anxious before my first session. I arrived at the Oncology Office and sat in the waiting room. I looked around and became painfully aware how much younger I was than the other patients. I was called into the chemotherapy room which was basically a room filled with chemotherapy chairs, chairs for visitors, a couple of televisions and a nurses station. Before being seated in the chemotherapy chair a lab technician drew blood to get a baseline of my blood levels. I would have a blood test every week—chemotherapy and off weeks—to monitor the impact of the drugs on my body. A nurse escorted me to a chair and the chemotherapy drip began. One down, seven to go!

For me treatment was about routine, consistency and comfort. The whole process lasted about three and a half hours. My nurse ensured that I always had the same corner chair which we dubbed "Cindy's Throne." This simple gesture minimized my anxiety by creating a sense of familiarity.

Every time I arrived, it looked like I was moving in. I brought my squooshy pillow, a cozy blanket, cozy socks, a Sudoku book (the best gift ever given to me), an iPod, a DVD player, sucking candy (critical for the port flushing as it often left a metallic taste in my mouth), magazines and bottles of water.

Team Cindy usually arrived with me or shortly there after. My family had "Team Cindy" t-shirts made and trekked in, bags in tow. They often camped out for the whole chemotherapy treatment. Friends would also stop by and visit, offering love and support and the occasional Starbucks!

I continued working during this time. I found that I only needed to take "Chemotherapy Thursday and Friday" off. I would, however, often work shorter days, and take naps mid day.

From talking to my cancer sisters, I knew that chemotherapy had a cumulative effect, meaning it would get harder with each treatment. I became to intimately know the cycle of feeling bad after chemotherapy and then slowly feeling better just before the next chemotherapy session. I felt the third treatment was the hardest because I started experiencing side effects like hot flashes, fuzziness, insomnia, bloating, and increased fatigue. By this point I had also lost all of my hair (head, legs, armpits, and pubic).

To prevent nausea I was given many different drugs. It was somewhat of a cocktail that would eventually keep my nausea at bay. The Friday after chemotherapy I received a Neulasta shot. Neulasta is a booster that helps stimulate white blood cells. For me, Saturday afternoons were the start of my down time. The chemotherapy usually made me feel fuzzy and the Neulasta injection created some joint aches.

After the first four chemotherapy treatments, my medications changed. I had heard from my cancer sisters, that the drug, Taxol, which I would take for the remaining treatments', was "easier." However, for me, I found the side effects to be much worse. During two of the Taxol treatments, my blood tests indicated that my red blood cells were lower than desired. To combat this I was given a drug which stimulates bone marrow and red blood cells. I also began experiencing Neuropathy (tingling/numbness) in my feet immediately after my first treatment. Arthritis and joint stiffness followed. By the third treatment, the Neuropathy began spreading to my hands and my Oncologist decided to forego the last session of Taxol.

Chemotherapy isn't easy. It, like cancer, is completely unique to the individual. No two people have the exact same experience. Still, it wasn't as bad as I had expected. Some good things also happened during chemotherapy. My skin looked radiant. I could also eat anything without my stomach getting upset. I still had sexual desire and felt like a sexual being despite everything.

Having loving friends, family and coworkers got me through chemotherapy with my spirit intact.

RADIATION

GINA

With months of chemotherapy and a mastectomy behind me, my wellness marathon continued. It was spring and I was recovering from a long winter. Peach fuzz, like that of a newborn covered my head. I continued to receive IV Herceptin treatments every three weeks, but the pathology from my mastectomy indicated a need for more treatment. Radiation was on deck. I met with a radiation oncologist to discuss my options. I was reluctant due to the possible complications. The doctor, a woman close to my age explained her recommendations and followed by saying that she was also a mother of young children. Her goal was for me to see my youngest son graduate from college. She understood! I made my decision, once again placing my life in someone else's hands. It was easier to do knowing that she had my best interest at heart. I trusted that she would plan my radiation and avoid damaging my heart and lungs. The thirty-three treatments began within weeks of my last chemotherapy, giving my body a little time to bounce back before a new assault began.

The mapping came first, a rather lengthy appointment during which the radiation fields are planned. The actual beam enters from different angles. The tissue expanders, part of my reconstruction, needed to be reduced in size. My plastic surgeon and my radiation oncologist worked together. Both were present and in one appointment, the size and shape of the expanders were altered to accommodate the radiation and my self esteem. They remained that way for the duration of the treatment. At this time, a series of little blue dot tattoos were placed on my chest to allow for consistent positioning. I was a little freaked out, wondering what they would throw at me next. Happily, I can report that the dots are so tiny that I never notice them. It was surreal as I lied on the cold table, chest exposed, arms up, trying not to move. The machines were intimidating but the techs were reassuring. Perhaps the most unnerving part of the whole process was my realization that as the technicians wrote on my chest with sharpie markers, I could not feel their hands on me. Wishing my mind was as numb as my chest, I went home, cried, took an Ativan and went to bed.

What's my time slot? The answer to that question would dictate my families schedule for the next seven weeks. It was my job to show up Monday-Friday at the same time every day. It was their job to help me get there. This would prove difficult when the kids began summer vacation in the middle of it all. Each appointment took about half an hour. Once a week I saw the doctor, which took an additional thirty minutes. Within a few days, I had it down to a science. The routine went like this: arrive at the hospital, drop the car with the valet, give a quick nod to the girls at the desk, grab a gown, quick change, wait in the holding area for the technician, hit the table, assume the position, watch the beams dance across my chest, back to the dressing room, apply cream, put on a loose top, and leave. This process has the potential of making a patient feel like they are in a "factory" setting. I found, however, that the technicians were very sensitive to this and were great at providing individual attention. They quickly became familiar with my life and soon were asking about my kids by name. It was comforting. On my last day of treatment, my new friends played graduation music and blew bubbles. They were truly happy for my accomplishment.

My chest wall and regional nodes were radiated. The final five treatments were a scar boost. I took great care of my skin and it held up remarkably well. I washed the area with gentle facial cleanser. I applied aloe gel, Alba cocoa butter lotion and traumeel gel, all of which I purchased at my local natural foods store. I only wore loose tops. I protected the area from the intense Florida sun with long sleeve cotton shirts or a surf top and of course sunscreen when appropriate.

Most bothersome was the pain that resided in my shoulder and between my shoulder blades. This sensation began almost immediately and became more intense as the weeks passed. It seemed that the awkward positioning of my arm during treatment, coupled with the radiation and the surgeries, was contributing to the problem. I remember struggling to lie still on the table at times because the pain was so intense. I ended up needing months of physical therapy to regain the range of motion in my shoulder and arm. Today I practice yoga and get massages to maintain my flexibility.

Like many other radiation patients, I also experienced fatigue which I managed by napping. Long term, I have a greater risk for lymphedema, a swelling of the arm.

Unfortunately, the radiation treatments complicated my reconstruction process as well. I experienced a firming of the skin in the radiated area. It was slow to heal during my expander/implant trade out surgery and quickly began to reject my new saline implant. The area became red and hot. Once I realized there was a problem I took off my surgery bra and began a light lymph drainage technique on that side, but it was too late. My plastic surgeon was forced to hospitalize me on Labor Day weekend. I was started on IV antibiotics that would continue for twelve days. He came to see me several times a day and on Sunday night at 11:00pm he walked into my hospital room, announced that he had just checked the O.R. and had decided to operate in the morning. I remember telling him I was afraid to have surgery on a holiday for fear of getting the "D" team doctors and nurses. He assured me that he had called in all the best people. But there was one more obstacle, what if the implant needed to be replaced? Where could we get one this late on a Sunday? The solution to this problem tickles me to this day. In a strange twist of fate, Jackie, one of my co-authors was scheduled for her TEI surgery later in the week. We were the same size. My surgeon would use Jackie's implant and get her another. He left the room saying "I'll see you first thing in the morning and remember not to eat anything after midnight."

The next day, as I was wheeled through the empty corridors of the hospital, I was remarkably calm thanks to my newly acquired meditation techniques. When I finally reached the operating room, I felt like the most special patient in the world. There I was, the only patient in a normally bustling facility and there they were, the "A" team. It was Labor Day. When I woke up, I had a drain in my radiated side and a loose dressing. I continued the light drainage massage on the effected area several times a day. This time, my body accepted the new implant that I affectionately call "Jackie." It sits up high and tight, just like she would want it to behave.

DEBBIE

As chemotherapy ended and the "chemo fog" began to lift, my radiation treatments began. Still on auto pilot, yet at a much less intense pace, I would get up, get dressed, put on my wig, drop the kids at school and head for the hospital. Once there, I would put on a gown, wait for my turn, remove my wig, receive the treatment (which took about five minutes after the initial visit), then retrace my steps towards home. I'd rest until school pick-up time and then have a few hours with my children until my husband came home from work.

Radiation therapy was much easier for me than chemotherapy. The physical body and joint pain and the feelings of being uncomfortable in my own skin were beginning to subside. I was starting to feel better. It felt good to be up and dressed in the morning and to be able to personally send my kids off to school. The technicians that administered my radiation were such a blessing. They were cheerful and compassionate. As intimidating as the machine is and as isolating as it feels to lie there in the darkened room alone, these two women did what they could to make it a personal experience and not seem so scary. Their kindheartedness will be with me for a long time.

One side effect was that my skin looked as if I had a bad sunburn. The last couple of treatments it actually felt burned too. My skin became uncomfortable to the touch. I remember thinking I had made it all the way to the end and being so disappointed that now my problems were going to begin. However, after the second or third boost treatment (the last week of my radiation treatment called for five treatments to the scar area only) my "burn" started going away. It never got worse than the bad sunburn. I was instructed to continue to put lotion on my skin for the next year and to be aware that I would probably be experiencing "effects" from the radiation for that amount of time as well. Some "healing" symptoms that I experienced were: isolated sharp pains in my breast, some swelling on and off and reduced flexibility in my arm and tightness around the scar tissue (some of the lack of flexibility was also attributed to the initial lumpectomy). Radiation also made me tired. It was as if it zapped my energy. Obviously I had not fully recovered from chemotherapy and now my body was being assaulted in yet another way. I made a conscious effort to rest as much as possible and to let my body focus on healing.

During my radiation treatment, I began going to physical therapy two to three times a week. As the "all over" body aches and pains from chemotherapy dissipated, the lack of flexibility and pain in my shoulder, arm and chest became more pronounced. Physical therapy was very beneficial for me. I was taught many great stretching exercises that I still do today. The treatment center had an on staff Lymphedema Specialist. Although I only had a few lymph nodes removed, developing Lymphedema during my lifetime is a very real concern for me. Given that there is no cure to reverse the effects of lymphedema, knowledge for prevention is vital. The specialist was able to share information about the lymphatic system, in terms that I would understand. In addition, she taught me how to maintain a healthy lymphatic system and preventative measures I could take.

I continue to see my Radiation Oncologist every six months. She is just as warm and approachable as her radiation team and I am very grateful for that.

DONNA

I made it through chemotherapy with several ups and downs. So I thought that radiation would be a walk in the park, boy, was I wrong! Many women who have a mastectomy on the cancerous breast don't need to have radiation. The doctors originally told me that I probably wouldn't need it either. After surgery they send your breast tissue off to the lab. It is bizarre to think that your body parts are being 'sent away' like they are going on vacation. But, my breasts were never coming back. After the lab did their dissection, they told me they found two more small tumors very close to my chest wall. I really didn't want to do radiation because it can cause complications with reconstruction. Scar tissue can build up around the implant and it can become harder and tighter to the chest. This contraction of the scar tissue can make the radiated breast with the implant higher than the other one. I decided to get a second opinion from another hospital. I was looking for a Doctor to tell me that I didn't need to have radiation, but I never found one. I was told I would have greater odds that the cancer would not return if I did radiation. I didn't want to regret it later. I wanted to do all things possible to beat the odds. Sign me up again! Off to radiation I went, skipping all the way.

I committed myself to going everyday for the next seven weeks. My first treatment was the hardest both physically and emotionally. When the technician came into the waiting room to get me I said "Just my luck!" My tech was a young good-looking guy! Why couldn't I have gotten a lady or even an old man? No guy had seen my breasts since my surgery. I now had to bear my virgin breasts, void of nipples, to him. He was the first. Now that's a first I'd like to forget! He was very professional and made me feel comfortable. There were two other young girls that also treated me. The radiation techs were the best. They were always pleasant, caring and in a positive mood. They made the trek out to the hospital everyday worthwhile.

The first radiation treatment takes about forty-five minutes. They have to set up the machine, map out the breast, take x-rays and tattoo you. I have to admit, this was my first tattoo. Okay, it doesn't qualify as a real tattoo. The cute, young tech put one dot in the middle of my chest and one on each side of my breasts. I guess we were bonding; he has forever left a "mark" on me. The tattoos are smaller than a freckle and they are used to align the machine to exact precision. As for the physical pain, I had to hold both of my arms behind my head for the entire treatment. Because I had joint pain as a result of the chemotherapy, I found it hard to hold that position for a long period of time. I just had to grin and bear it.

During the whole breast cancer experience, you are flashing your breasts to so many doctors that you just don't care anymore. It's like these new "ta-ta's" are not a part of your body. They feel like foreign objects, two mounds that I bought at the hospital. The implants even come with a serial number and a warranty, go figure.

I started out doing real well with my radiation treatments for the first five weeks. Then I developed a really bad burn, it seemed to come out of nowhere. It is important to radiate the skin and muscle area of the breast. I thought that I would breeze through radiation because I have olive Italian skin. I tan easily and rarely burn. The radiologist told me that this is a myth. People with fair skin can do real well and vice versa, but burn I did!

I have implants so the radiation technician put a device called a Bollis on me. The bollis is used to trick the machine to think that you have thicker skin. By doing this, it keeps more of the radiation on the surface skin and muscle. This thick, flexible piece of plastic was placed on my breast every other day. I am not sure but wonder if the bollis may have exacerbated my burns.

It all started with a group of small blisters by my underarm and the sensitive skin underneath of my breast where the sun never shines. The actual breast was OK, except for the brown discoloration from the burn. The problem was the skin surrounding the breast area that took the brunt of it. The blisters were very itchy. It had that feeling of when you itch something, it feels better for a moment, and then the itch comes back instantly with a fury. One morning I awoke in a frenzy, I was so consumed with itch that I couldn't see straight. I went directly to the Radiation Center to see the doctor without an appointment. With Darci's help, I was able to see the doctor right away.

I left with two prescriptions; one for a medicated cream and the other was for an antihistamine. I left the doctor's office all agitated and was speeding to the pharmacy to fill my prescriptions. The morning didn't start off too good and didn't get any better. I was pulled over by a cop for speeding. Now, this was the perfect opportunity to pull out the "Cancer Card", but I didn't. At this point, I was so over everything that I didn't care at the time. When the cop came back to the car to give me the ticket he saw a flyer on my passenger's side seat that was for a lecture on cancer for Dealing with Fatigue. He asked me if I had cancer and I said "yes". Then he goes on to tell me that he had testicular cancer when he was younger. How strange? Was this supposed to make me feel better about getting a ticket? Maybe he could have ripped up the ticket, but no such luck for me. I got hit while I was down. Note to readers, this was the perfect opportunity to pull out the "Cancer Card"; you have it, so use it when necessary!

Back to the burn, within two days the medications made me feel so much better. It was at this time that the blisters opened and I had six inches of an open wound/burn under my left breast. The medicated cream was applied for another week. It felt good when first applied, but as it caked-up and dried out it would crack and become very painful if I moved the wrong way. I was very uneasy about continuing treatments. It just didn't seem normal or safe to radiate an open wound. Having come this far, I couldn't quit now. I constantly questioned this treatment to my doctor. She finally said that she wanted to get in just a few more rounds of treatment. There is a minimum amount of radiation that they believe needs to be achieved before stopping treatment. The Bollis was removed from the treatment regime once the burn reared its ugly head. At the end, I had to do five

Booster treatments that focused just on the incision area of the breast. If the cancer was to return, it usually comes back at the incision area.

Aside from the shoulder joint pain, the actual two minutes of radiation treatments were painless and a piece of cake. Everyday I was in and out of the clinic within fifteen minutes. The radiation room is kept very cold, if I had nipples, they would have been hard! All throughout the seven weeks of treatment, I had to apply creams and moisturizers daily. The recommended cream is very thick and greasy. I was not able to wear a bra due to the burn. I made sure I put the greasy cream on at night with an old t-shirt. The cream would actually stain the shirt. I would apply the other creamy moisturizer throughout the day.

One of the most exhausting things about radiation is getting there everyday and trying to be on time. I had to rush thru traffic and this was very stressful. In addition to that, I had to make sure I didn't schedule any business meetings around my treatment times. I felt like a slave to the schedule. I couldn't go on vacations during this time, and after chemotherapy, I desperately needed one!

HORMONAL THERAPY

"While I am taking this drug, I cannot have children. Fearing that chemo-therapy would put me into permanent menopause, my husband and I went to a fertility specialist before I had surgery and chemotherapy. He used a new technique to stimulate my ovaries while keeping my estrogen levels low. We then had embryos made and frozen. We now have three embryos waiting to be born!'

—Tamara

TAMARA

I was placed on Tamoxifen, a drug that lowers estrogen levels in your body, because my tumor was estrogen positive. I have to take it for five years. Side effects that I have noticed are: vaginal dryness and thinning of the vaginal lining, problems with my eyes, mood swings, and an increase in appetite. Because I have to take this pill for so long, I have been struggling to find ways to make these issues bearable.

Vaginal dryness results from the lack of estrogen and makes it extremely hard to have sex. I was constantly itchy and burning and even had a vaginal tear. My oncologist and gynecologist agreed that I could use a low estrogen vaginal cream two times a week. I use Premarin, but there are also others available. I have seen a very big improvement with this. My husband is thrilled!

My eyes became extremely dry and irritated. I went to my eye doctor and discovered that I had corneal abrasions. They are treated with steroid drops and eye exams every six months.

I also experienced a huge increase in appetite. I was hungry 24 hours a day and began to gain weight again. I was able to get it off and keep it off by working out every other day, doing toning exercises and weight lifting followed by cardiovas-cular exercises. In addition, I joined Jenny Craig. I am still very hungry, but being on a strict diet has helped me maintain my weight. I plan to stay on this diet until I am done with the Tamoxifen.

One of the most troubling side effects for me is the mood swings. I felt better when I began taking a light dose anti-depressant. I feel more in control and happy.

While I am taking Tamoxifen, I cannot have children. Fearing that chemo-therapy would put me into permanent menopause, my husband and I went to a fertility specialist before I had surgery and chemotherapy. He used a new technique to stimulate my ovaries while keeping my estrogen levels low. We then had embryos made and frozen. We now have three embryos waiting to be born!

My husband and I are newly married and we need time to pull our lives back together. We now have five years to do that. I also came out of menopause and restarted my cycles so we can try to have children naturally if the embryos don't take.

JACKIE

Tamoxifen is an important part of my fight against breast cancer, especially in preventing a reoccurrence. As much as I dislike the side effects I still take it everyday.

The most troublesome side effect I experience is mood swings. There is no way to predict when one will hit me and it is very unsettling to feel so out of control. The only thing that I feel that helps my unfavorable disposition is exercise. I always feel better and more in control of myself when I work out regularly. It is part of my daily routine.

I am thankful there is a medicine like Tamoxifen available to me. So, I grin and bear it and literally, take my medicine!

DEBBIE

Because of the fact that I had Estrogen Positive breast cancer, was 37 years old and premenopausal, my Oncologist recommended a daily dose of Tamoxifen for approximately five years. The "approximately" is unique to my situation because in addition to a lumpectomy, chemotherapy and radiation, I also participated in a study where I was given an injection of the drug Triptorelin every 28 days. This medicine "shut down" my ovaries, removing a major supplier of estrogen for my body. I began the study at the same time that I started chemotherapy. I continued to receive an injection every 28 days until I had my ovaries removed which was about two months after I completed my radiation treatments.

My Oncologist now monitors me to determine when I will be considered "post" menopausal. The chemotherapy, Triptorelin injections and the removal of my ovaries have started the process. Once I am post menopausal, I will be switched to another Estrogen blocking drug that is better suited for my needs.

DONNA

I am currently on the drug Tamoxifen and will continue to take it everyday for five years. Tamoxifen is to help prevent a reoccurrence of breast cancer. Initially I was hesitant to take it when I finished chemotherapy and radiation treatment because of some of the side effects I heard may occur from its use. I decided I need to do all things possible to help prevent a reoccurrence. I don't want to regret any decision that I made. I have to live with myself and be at peace about it. God forbid the cancer comes back! At least know that I did all I could.

ADDITIONAL THERAPY

DEBBIE

In addition to chemotherapy, radiation and hormonal therapy, I chose to have my ovaries removed. Although I did not test positive for any of the known breast cancer genes, I still had an increased risk of ovarian cancer because I had been diagnosed with breast cancer under the age of 40.

At the start of my chemotherapy, I also began participating in a study that provided me with a drug named Triptorelin. Its primary function was to shut down my ovaries, to stop the production of estrogen. This act was beneficial for me because my breast cancer was fueled by estrogen. (I was diagnosed with estrogen positive breast cancer). The drug is received via an injection every 28 days. I was "artificially" put into menopause due to my chemotherapy treatments and the Triptorelin injections.

Prior to my breast cancer diagnosis, my husband and I had discussed not having anymore children. We already had two amazing children and were content with the dynamics of our family. This decision, along with the benefits I would receive from eliminating a major source of estrogen, made my decision to remove my ovaries as a preventative measure valid in my eyes and in the opinions of my doctors.

The procedure was done laproscopically by my OBGYN as an out-patient procedure.

TAMARA

My tumors were HER2 positive, so I received Herceptin, a new drug given intravenously to target directly the HER2 receptor and thereby kill all the cancer cells. I received these treatments every three weeks for a full year. At first it wasn't so bad. My hair was able to grow back, I didn't get nauseous or sick like with the other drugs. I felt a little weird for a few hours after treatment but then I would snap out of it.

It took about 90 minutes to administer because it made me woozy if given faster. I would go in with a bag full of stuff. I had my snacks (the Herceptin tastes bad), water, a good book and my ipod. I would grab a blanket and make myself comfy. In my chemotherapy room they even had a little TV over each chair, which made it more interesting.

Towards the end, this drug had a cumulative type affect. The last three treatments were very hard. Instead of feeling weird for a few hours, I would feel bloated, have heartburn, and be completely mentally fuzzy for days. I would go home, wander from room to room trying to remember what I was doing. The worst was the depression. I would feel a "black cloud" enveloping me within hours of the treatment. I had severe mood swings.

I feel fortunate to have received Herceptin, since it was just approved for general use, but I do believe the doctors should tell us a little more about the side effects. I felt that they led me to believe that there were practically none. Granted, you don't lose your hair and you are not extremely nauseous, but there are still side effects that are cumulative and disturbing to your everyday life. You feel as though you are moving on and getting better (hair growing back, etc.) but with each successive treatment I felt worse for a longer period of time. Although side effects may not be as severe in all cancer patients, I think we should be warned that they can occur so that we know what to expect. About three weeks after my last Herceptin treatment, my depression and wild mood swings were reduced to recognizable PMS.

JACKIE

Another drug that was prescribed to me was Herceptin. I took it every three weeks for one year after finishing my chemotherapy. Fortunately, the Herceptin did not affect my hair re-growth and it did not seem as toxic as my chemotherapy medications. Still, the Herceptin was administered through my port, just as the chemotherapy drugs. There were preparation drugs given first and side effects after. Psychologically, it was sometimes difficult preparing myself for the next treatment.

Some experiences I had were feeling as if I was in a fog, lacking energy, and mood swings. Sometimes I also felt depressed. The depression was probably a combination of the medicine and having to return to the chemotherapy treatment center to receive it. It was also difficult to see all the new faces, young and old, over the course of the year. It would especially affect me when I saw someone there for their first time. It was very difficult to go to those treatment sessions.

I am so thankful for my family and friends who gave me the strength to get there each time. They helped me to have the courage I needed to do something so difficult, but necessary.

ALTERNATIVE THERAPY

CINDY

In conjunction with my chemotherapy, I added acupuncture after my second treatment. I found that it helped alleviate some mild soreness that I was experiencing and helped me feel relaxed. It also seemed to minimize some of the "chemo fog" I often felt during the treatments.

I also decided to see a social worker weekly. Sherri (who had conducted the healing circle) had known me for a few years and provided a safe haven where I could discuss everything I was thinking and feeling in a safe, private environment. It was nice to have an objective resource who listened as I talked about my fears, anger, insecurity, and any other emotion that crept up during the treatment process. I found that having Sherri proved particularly invaluable AFTER chemotherapy had ended and I started the slow journey back to my "new normal".

Many therapists feel that going through a cancer experience can lead to post traumatic stress symptoms. I know that I personally rode a very intense roller coaster of emotions after my treatments were over. I found having a constant source support and dialogue from Sherri was invaluable for me. We talked about everything. The topics ranged from my ability and desire to have children in the future, the role that my BRCA 1 status plays in my life, my self image, emotional highs and lows, anger management and coping skills after chemotherapy, sexuality, relationships, living as a cancer survivor, fear of a recurrence, redefining my sense of self and a myriad of subjects that came and went and sometimes came back again in the months after my treatment ended.

DONNA

I started to receive acupuncture at the say time that I started chemotherapy. I had little knowledge of acupuncture and had never tried it before. Now that I was diagnosed with cancer, I was open to almost any alternative treatments to help me along the way. I was told it could help with some of the side effects from chemotherapy. You didn't have to twist my arm, I was there. I would welcome anything that would help me get through chemotherapy. I went once a week all the way through my chemotherapy treatments and radiation.

When I first started going I was in good health and did not have any ailments at the time. As the chemotherapy progressed, so did the side effects. I was treated for several different side effects each time. I really had nothing to judge from, so it is hard to say if acupuncture really worked. My side effects may have been worse if I didn't do acupuncture, I will never know. Overall, it is a very relaxing treatment. I found that is relieved a lot of stress and calmed me down. Don't believe people when they say, "the needles are so tiny, you can't feel them." I felt them alright! It's like they were digging to China! They twist the needle in until it hits a nerve, then they know it's deep enough and working. The good thing is that the needles don't hurt coming out. I had a team of two young ladies working on me each visit. They are a great team and some hip chicks and they always made me laugh which is great medicine. I looked forward to going each week.

We hope you are feeling connected and have the sense that you are not alone. It is important to remember that everyone's experience is different. We each reacted differently to each drug, some having more side effects than others. We all had a variety of methods for coping and finding comfort. Find what makes each day easier for you and what will get you to that next chemotherapy appointment and focus on it.

Your doctors are helping you to fight breast cancer with the best treatments available. It is strong medicine, and it is part of your armaments to fight your cancer. This is your opportunity to let your cancer know that it's not going to defeat you.

THE MEDICAL TEAM:

RADIATION ONCOLOGIST

RASHMI BENDA, MD

Dr. Rashmi Benda, M.D. is a board Certified Radiation Oncologist. She received her medical degree from the University Of Miami School Of Medicine in 1994. She completed her internship at the Sinai Hospital of Detroit in 1995 and her residency in Radiation Oncology at Wayne State University in 1998.

She has since held faculty positions at Loyola University Cancer Center in Illinois and University of Florida. She has an interest and expertise in Breast Cancer. She was the Co-Director of the Breast Cancer Center at Loyola. She developed new clinical programs including Breast IMRT as well as Active Breathing Control at University of Florida.

She has also been involved in research as a reviewer for scientific journals and American Society of Therapeutic Radiology and Oncology. She has also published several peer-reviewed papers and book chapters. She has not only presented papers at national and international meetings, but also enjoys giving community lectures.

She is currently practicing at the Boca Raton Community Hospital, in Florida. Dr. Benda is heavily involved with the breast cancer program. She is the Co-Director of their breast multi-modality clinic for breast cancer patients that she was instrumental in launching.

THE ROLE OF RADIATION AS PART OF BREAST CANCER TREATMENT

Radiation is recommended routinely after a lumpectomy. This allows a woman to preserve her breast without compromising her recurrence rate or survival. Studies looking at patients with very favorable cancers also show a benefit to radiation after a lumpectomy. Sometimes, radiation is also recommended after a mastectomy. In women with four or more lymph nodes or tumor greater than five centimeters radiation is strongly recommended. Although, there is convincing data that women with any positive lymph nodes may benefit from post-mastectomy radiation. The benefit in decreased local recurrence translates into a survival benefit 10 to 15 years later. Close or positive margins after a mastectomy also warrant radiation.

THE RADIATION PROCESS

Radiation is a local treatment. The team involved in ensuring proper delivery of radiation consists of a Radiation Oncologist, nurses, therapists (they set you up on a daily basis for treatment), dosimetrist (most of their work is done behind the scenes helping the radiation oncologist customize the radiation to each patient), and physicist (is responsible for proper functioning of the machines which includes periodic calibration. The physicist also oversees the therapists and the dosimetrists.)

When a patient is ready to begin radiation the process starts with a CT simulation. A CT scan is obtained in the treatment position (usually with one or both arms above the head, supported by a mold or beast board). Markers are placed on the skin as a guide for certain anatomic landmarks that may not be easily visible on CT. At the end of the simulation process, the patient leaves with a few tattoos that are smaller than most freckles, but permanent. The CT images are then transferred to the treatment planning computers. The radiation oncologist then outlines the radiation targets (tumor bed, breast, lymph nodes, etc.) and the avoidance structures (lung, heart). With the help of a dosimetrist an ideal plan best suited for the individual patient is achieved. In some cases this may be a 3D plan while in other cases it is an IMRT (Intensity modulated radiation therapy) plan is obtained. Once the ideal plan is obtained this information is transferred to the treatment machines. The radiation therapists then use this information to setup the patient and take measurements as well as films that are approved by the physician to ensure proper treatment delivery.

The treating physician monitors the patient on a weekly basis by checking the films taken on the machine and the patient's symptoms. If needed, the plan can be altered based on the symptoms.

The first follow-up visit 4–6 weeks after treatment is to ensure resolution of any symptoms during the course of treatment and establish a long term follow-up plan including imaging as well as periodic physical exams.

A PERSONAL NOTE FROM THE DOCTOR

I went to medical school like a lot of young girls wanting to be a pediatrician. During my pediatric rotation, I realized I loved to play with kids, but did not feel an academic challenge. I recalled how I had been fascinated by the patho-physiology of cancer. This led me to explore medical oncology, the field everyone thinks of when they think of cancer. Two weeks of rotating through medical oncology, I still felt no chemistry. It wasn't as if I was looking to marry my specialty, or was I?

After a month of surgical oncology, I thought I knew what I wanted to do for the rest of my life.

Around that same time, a dear friend whose father is a medical physicist recommended I explore Radiation Oncology. Push buttons and zap people? How challenging could that be? Still, I let myself get talked into a rotation in radiation oncology. It turned out to be amazing. I had found my passion. Yes, I would spend time seeing patients, and be challenged with the pathological and technical aspects of treatment planning. I have been able to continue my learning through my patients, but I have also been fortunate enough to share my knowledge with others taking care of breast cancer patients through publications and lectures.

As routine as every profession becomes, I continue to be challenged everyday. My challenges range from reaching the decision to radiate, encouraging someone to continue treatment despite the side effects and hassle of daily treatments, and most difficult of all, helping women cope with the diagnosis. I've made several patients cry by just asking, "How are you coping?"On a positive note, it is encouraging to see patients wanting to be involved in their care. I love to arm my patients with the data that empowers them with the knowledge to make their own decisions. I commend my patients for being proactive in their care. I encourage second opinions. I share with my patients that medicine is an art as well as science. Physicians may vary in their recommendations and still be within the guidelines.

When I tell people what I do, they usually offer me pity. "That must be so hard!" How do you deal with it?" "Do you take stress home?" The answer to all of these questions is, yes! But, there are many more rewards than disappointments in my field. I celebrate every victory; from the healing of radiation side effects to knowing that the radiation has improved someone's chance of remaining cancer-free. My rewards are not always immediate, but every study that reports improvement in survival in those who had radiation puts a smile on my face. To know that now a woman has a better chance of being there for her children's graduations, weddings and all other important events in their lives. I cannot think of anything I would rather do! There are also those whose disease I cannot cure, but the joy I feel when their quality of life is improved is beyond words.

Why I chose this field, I'm asked. Even on my worst day when I ask myself that question, my patient's remind me why and they don't even know it! My days are as challenging as they are rewarding.

LYMPHEDEMA

Susan Lanham, PT/CLT

Susan is a physical therapist who has been in practice for 28 years. She received a BS and Certificate in Physical Therapy from Simmons College in Boston, MA and Certification in treatment of lymphedema from Lerner Lymphedema Services Academy. She is currently a senior physical therapist specializing in treatment of lymphedema at the Davis Therapy Center of Boca Raton Community Hospital.

LYMPHEDEMA

Lymphedema is a potential side effect of breast cancer treatment affecting on average 25% of patients. While sentinel node biopsy is now used whenever possible and has a much lower incidence of lymphedema, approximately 3–7%, lymphedema is still a concern for breast cancer survivors and can be a troubling reminder of the disease they are trying to put behind them.

Some common questions asked are: Should I be concerned about lymphedema? What is it? What are my risks? Can it be prevented? If I get lymphedema can it be treated and what is the treatment? This chapter will attempt to answer these questions and give you some general guidelines for lymphedema prevention. Because each person's medical history and risk factors are unique you must discuss your concerns as soon as you have them with the members of your cancer care team.

WHAT IS LYMPHEDEMA AND WHY MAY IT OCCUR AFTER TREATMENT FOR BREAST CANCER?

Lymphedema is the swelling of a body part due to an accumulation of lymph fluid. In the breast cancer patient this may occur due to surgical removal of lymph nodes in the under arm and/or radiation therapy to the same area. Swelling may occur in the arm, hand, breast or chest wall on the affected side.

The lymphatic system is part of your circulatory system. It consists of a one-way network of vessels returning fluid from the interstitium (spaces between the cells) back to the central circulatory system. Lymph is comprised of water and larger particles including proteins, fats, cell debris and foreign particles such as bacteria. Lymph nodes are located more centrally in the body and their job is to filter and concentrate the lymph. The lymphatic system also plays an important roll in your immunity by producing cells which fight infection.

Removal of lymph nodes in the underarm area (axiliary lymph node dissection) usually accompanies mastectomy or lumpectomy. Axillary node dissection is a valued staging procedure for breast cancer with findings influencing clinical decision making and helping predict recurrence risk and survival. Unfortunately it has possible complications which may include numbness, pain, limited shoulder motion and lymphedema. Sentinel node biopsy, as less invasive staging procedure, is now used whenever possible and carries less risk.

In summary the risk of developing lymphedema is associated with axillary node dissection, especially if node dissection is extensive, radiation therapy to the axilla and the risk increases with the combination of these. It is best to discuss your individual risk for lymphedema with your cancer care physicians and surgeons.

LYMPHEDEMA SYMPTOMS/WHAT TO LOOK FOR

Visible swelling of the arm, hand, breast or chest wall

Sensation of tightness, pressure, heaviness, aching or pulling in the arm

Sensation of fullness in the underarm

Sleeves and jewelry may feel tight

Arm may feel firm to the touch

Symptoms of lymphedema may develop soon after treatment or many years later. Most women who develop lymphedema do so within the first 4 years after treatment.

Please note that it is usual to have some swelling in the area of your surgery immediately after surgery. This is part of the healing process and should subside over the next several months.

LYMPHEDEMA RISK REDUCTION

While it has not been proven that you can prevent lymphedema, you may reduce your risk by following these guidelines.

Wear a compression sleeve and glove for exercise, flying and repetitive arm tasks.

A class 1, (20–30 mmHg compression) sleeve and glove are recommended. These may be obtained from a medical supply properly trained in compression garment fitting or your physical therapist. You will need a doctor's prescription.

Avoid trauma/injury to the at risk quadrant.

Avoid any breaks in the skin. No injections, no blood drawn in the at risk arm. Use care when shaving underarms. Avoid cutting cuticles during nail care. If you notice a break in your skin, wash the area with soap and running water, apply antibacterial ointment and observe the area for signs of infection.

Know the signs of infection (redness, swelling, heat, fever). Call your doctor immediately if you suspect an infection. Usually these require prescription antibiotics.

Wear gloves for gardening, household cleaning and handling harsh cleansers.

Avoid temperature extremes. Saunas, hot tubs not recommended. Protect yourself from the sun with sun block and/or protective clothing.

Avoid unnecessary weight gain. Excess weight increases the demands on the tissue and circulatory system.

Avoid constriction of the at risk arm. No blood pressure cuffs on that side. Avoid tight jewelry, tight watch straps and shoulder bags.

Elevated your at risk arm and pump your hand periodically. This encourages circulatory return.

Daily self-massage. This is taught by a therapist certified in lymphedema treatment. If you have not had proper training in self massage, using light upward strokes on the at risk extremity when soaping in the shower or applying your body lotion is recommended.

Aquatic exercise and swimming are beneficial. Check with your doctor first especially if you have not yet completed chemotherapy or radiation therapy or breast reconstruction. Water exercise is not recommended if you have open wounds due to risk of infection and delayed wound healing.

Diaphragmatic breathing or "belly breathing" is beneficial as it encourages circulatory return from the extremities. ~Seven deep breaths, once an hour are recommended. Do not deep breath to the point of lightheadedness.

LYMPHEDEMA TREATMENT

To arrange consultation or treatment you will first need a prescription from a doctor on your cancer care team.

Breast cancer patients who do not have lymphedema but are at risk may schedule an evaluation and individual educational session with a therapist specializing in lymphedema treatment.

The treatment for those who have lymphedema is called Complete Decongestive Physical Therapy (CDP).

It has 4 components:

Manual Lymph Drainage (MLD) is a gentle massage which stimulates lymph flow and redirects edema to normally functioning lymphatic vessels.

Compression Bandaging composed of low elastic, multi-layer, cotton bandages are applied to the affected limb to enhance muscle pumping action and prevent re-accumulation of edema. Those with mild edema may not need to bandage.

Therapeutic Exercises are performed with compression bandages or compression garments in place to improve lymphatic circulation as well as muscle tone. Individual advice about what sort of exercises may be beneficial versus aggravating is also given.

Education in self-management including proper skin care, edema prevention and control, self bandaging if necessary, self-massage, exercise and appropriate use of compression garments is essential for effective long term management of lymphedema.

COMPRESSION SLEEVES AND GLOVES

Compression sleeves and gloves are elastic garments which are worn to prevent lymphedema or to maintain the edema reduction achieved with treatment (CDP). They may be purchased at a medical supply store and must be properly fitted by a certified fitter. You will need a prescription from the doctor. Your doctor or physical therapist can recommend a reliable medical supply. Most people fit into off-the-shelf garments, but custom garments are available.

If you are at risk for and trying to prevent lymphedema it is recommended you wear a 20–30mmHg compression sleeve and possibly a glove when you exercise, when you fly and when you are performing repetitive arm tasks.

If you have lymphedema and have had treatment your therapist will recommend a compression garment and wearing schedule. Daily wearing of compression garments is typically recommended until the condition settles. Then you should wear the garments for exercise, flying and repetitive arm tasks. Consult your therapist with any questions.

Do not sleep in the compression garments. Special night garments or compression bandages may be recommended for patients with lymphedema who need night compression.

EXERCISE AND LYMPHEDEMA

Specific guidelines for exercise are probably better addressed by your doctor and physical therapist on a case by case basis. In general most experts agree that aquatic exercise is the most beneficial for lymphedema as the water has a compressive and gentle massaging effect. Cooler water temperatures are best.

Gentle, rhythmic exercise such as tai chi, yoga and Pilates are recommended. Low impact aerobics or gentle bouncing on a trampoline is also helpful.

Exercises that involve heavy weight lifting, sustained isometrics or repetitive arm swinging are riskier for the following reasons. With lifting heavier weights there is increased work load and possible micro-trauma to the target muscles. This increases circulation to the arm which may then have some difficulty exiting the arm due to lower lymphatic capacity. With sustained isometrics (gripping) there is an increase in muscle work load but a decrease in the muscle pumping action which aids in circulatory return. The arm swinging motion which is part of sports like tennis, racquet ball and, to a lesser extent, golf has a centrifugal effect on the arm and may tend to push fluid into the hand. Some sports include elements of lifting, gripping and swinging and these are considered higher risk activities.

So, does this mean you should not participate in these sports? No. Consider your level of risk, discuss it with your doctor and therapist, wear a compression sleeve and glove when you exercise and resume these activities slowly.

USEFUL WEBSITES

National Lymphedema Network (NLN) www.lymphnet.org

The Susan G. Komen Breast Foundation www.komen.org

American Cancer Society www.cancer.org

BOOKS

Lymphedema, A Breast Cancer Patient's Guide to Prevention and Healing by Jeannie Burt and Gwen White, 1999. ISBN 0-897932641

Lymphedema: Understanding and Managing Lymphedema After Cancer, 2006. ISBN 0944235-56-5

Living Well with Lymphedema by Ann Erlich, Alma Vinje-Harrewijn, Elizabeth McMahon, 2005. ISBN 0-9764806-1-1

CHAPTER FIVE

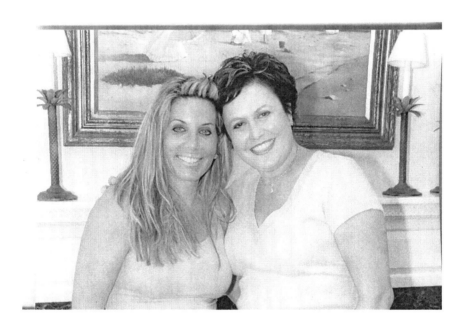

FEELING BEAUTIFUL

"I always tried to look my best, even when I felt my worst. I was still a young sexy attractive female even though I looked different. I resolved to be the best looking cancer patient that I could be. Most people look at me now and have no idea that I had cancer or if they do, they say, "Wow, it's not so bad to get breast cancer." I think that's pretty cool."

—*Tamara*

For the majority of women diagnosed with breast cancer, especially young women, the reality of being diagnosed with breast cancer starts to sink in when the oncologist says, "During your treatment, you will lose your hair." We have yet to meet a young cancer survivor that was not devastated by those words. The only words harder to hear are: "its only hair" and "it will grow back". Of course it will grow back and we know that is the least of our problems.

In today's society, many wigs are stylish and natural looking. They are easier to care for than natural hair. Bald is beautiful and bandanas are worn everywhere. Still, looking good and feeling good often go hand in hand. For most women, how can you look good and feel good about yourself if you are a woman with no hair?

This is a very special part of the book for us. It is the topic doctors don't elaborate on, friends and families don't want to bring up, and there is very little in books or on the internet about it. Yet it is on a young breast cancer patient's mind twenty-four hours a day.

The following is your validation.

IT'S ONLY HAIR, IT WILL GROW BACK

*"Hair is part of your identity. When people heard that I had breast cancer,
I felt like I was on display. Everyone was looking at me to see if I was ok and
to see how cancer had affected me. Losing my hair was one of the most difficult things about having breast cancer."*

—*Jackie*

JACKIE

Hair is part of your identity. When people heard that I had breast cancer, I felt
like I was on display. Everyone was looking at me to see if I was ok and to see
how cancer had affected me. Losing my hair was one of the most difficult things
about having breast cancer.

I was embarrassed about having to wear a wig. I had always had long beautiful
hair. It was one of the things I liked most about my appearance. I wasn't sure
how I was going to deal with hair loss and the effects of chemotherapy.

Thank goodness for my teenagers. Adolescents and their naturally heightened
awareness of one's appearance were my saving grace. My kids knew just where to
get a wig. (Our mall actually had a great kiosk.) They were my biggest critics. I
knew that if they were approving, I must look ok. Still, it took a lot of getting
used to. As I began feeling more comfortable around family and friends I went
everywhere wearing my wig. It became my security blanket. I went out, went to
work and even ran four miles for exercise everyday while wearing it.

Nonetheless, I couldn't wait for chemotherapy to be over so my hair would
begin to grow back. As treatment ended, my daily "hair checks" began. Unfortunately it takes much longer for your hair to grow back, than it did to fall out.
First, I was waiting for my head to be fully covered. Then, as much as I wanted to
stop wearing my wig, how could I? I had a head full of hair, but it was only a half
an inch long! I had lived my entire life with long hair; it was part of how I identified myself. My feelings of being on display were creeping up on me again. I
wanted to move on. I wanted to move past being a "cancer patient", but how
could I with such a drastic change in hair style? Such a dramatic change in my
identity.

I continued to wear my wig until my hair was long enough for hair extensions
(about six months). Then, after the many hours it takes to put the extensions in,
I was able to move on from the wig. My hair looked beautiful. The extensions
would give my hair the chance to grow in without the uncomfortable wig cover-

ing it. I could go to sleep and wake up with "hair" like I had been used to my whole life. The extensions gave me more freedom and confidence.

The day after getting my new hair, I took my wigs to the facilitator of our support group. I hope they can give someone else the same security they provided me. Most importantly, I am thankful to be cancer free and alive. But, as a woman, you know how "a good hair day" makes you feel!

CINDY

The idea of losing my hair was the scariest, most agonizing part of my Cancer treatment. I've always been a "lucky hair girl." I had relatively thick hair that basically did whatever I wanted. I could wear it straight, I could wear it wavy. I wore bangs, I grew it out. I colored it from brown, to blonde to auburn.

People asked me why losing my hair bothered my more than losing my breasts. Everybody said "it will grow back." But for some reason, the external image, the public persona I associated with myself always included my hair. In my own mind, I could hide my boobs under clothing, with bras etc. But my bald head would scream "Cancer" to the world and that wasn't my choice.

DONNA

If one more person says, "It's only hair, it'll grow back," I WILL scream! The first thing I asked my surgeon when he told me I would need chemotherapy was "Will I lose my hair?" Unfortunately, he said "yes"!

Losing my hair was a big concern to me. The big hang-up was fear of the unknown. Most women have never experienced hair loss. Our hair is our crown that we wear out everyday. We've all had bad hair days but few of us know what it is like to have a no hair day. My hair reached to the middle of my back before I found out I had breast cancer. I decided to cut my hair shoulder length before surgery to help ease the pain of cutting it all off at once.

Just like clockwork, around two weeks after my first chemotherapy treatment, I started to lose some of my hair. If I would pull on a small cluster of hair it would come out without putting up a fight. When I would take a shower, I would have a lot of hair in my hands and on the shower floor. I would have to pick the hair up off of the shower floor and throw it out. It was definitely too much hair to go down the drain with out clogging it. That grossed me out the most. So, I decided to go to the salon and have my head shaved. I was going to control the situation before it controlled me. I thought that I was going to cry when I had it shaved, but I didn't, it was quite the opposite. The hair stylist had me turned away from the mirror while he went to town with the hair clippers. I brought along my girlfriend and parents for moral support. When he was done, he spun me around and I blurted out a scream followed by loads of laughter! It was a shock to see myself bald. I looked like I was ready to go into the Army. It felt really neat to touch my head! The hair stylist then put my wig on, the wig that I bought before surgery, and proceeded to cut it and thin it out.

My "wiggy" thoughts could comprise an entire chapter. To be quite honest, I felt like an imposter. Even though my wig was thinned out and styled, it was much "hairier" than my real hair. I thought I looked like a TV anchorwoman with a plastic looking perfectly styled hairdo.

One of the perks of having breast cancer is that I could get ready in the morning in fifteen minutes! It takes only one minute to throw on the wig, fluff it into place, and walah, I was ready to go. Another perk is that you can have as many wigs as you want to experiment with hair colors and styles. You can just pick the wig that matches your mood for the day and off you go.

I must admit at times I felt like I was wearing a muskrat on my head. It took a long time to get used to wearing it. I was always looking into a mirror or my reflection in the window to see if my hair was out of place. The down side is that you can't "feel" if your hair is messed up. I was self conscious about my wig and I constantly wondered if people that didn't know me could tell it was a wig. I received many compliments on the color of it. I had more compliments on my wig than my real hair. Hmm, maybe that should tell me something about my old hair! Note to self, don't go back to the same color and style again.

I am hot-blooded Italian and wearing the wig just made me hotter. I'm not talking looks, but temperature! The wig can get very hot. To top it off, I would get hot flashes from the chemotherapy and I would be tempted to whip the wig off in public! But I couldn't, I didn't have the nerve to do it, but wish I did. It would be worth seeing the reaction on people's faces.

One thing that I always wondered about was when people would say that my wig "looks real" and that they "would have never known it if I didn't tell them". I wish I had a dollar for every time I heard that line. Did they really think that? Were they just trying to be nice? I can spot a muskrat from a mile away, couldn't they? I never did the "scarf look" it's just wasn't me. I felt like if I wore a scarf it would just draw attention to me and read like a billboard "I have cancer!" I was not interested in advertising it.

GINA

I asked my husband what it was like when I was bald and he said "I was sad every day, not for me but for you because I know how much it affected you." He was right, it made me sad and it did bother me, a lot. It served as a constant reminder that I was cancer patient. Even on the days when I felt like my old self, a glance in the mirror or any reflective surface would bring the reality of my situation rushing back.

I wonder if the doctors who are charged with delivering the diagnosis of cancer are surprised when patients ask first "Am I going to die?" followed immediately by "Am I going to lose my hair?" Hair seems so insignificant in the grand scheme of things. It wasn't until I lost mine that I realized our culture is obsessed with hair. The amount of money and time we spend on at times seems ridiculous.

From the start I decided to be up front with my children about my illness. The night I told my 5 year old that my medicine was going to make my hair fall out, he looked at me with bewilderment. He was having trouble comprehending. "You mean all your hair? You'll be bald?" he asked. Then he burst into tears and I hadn't expected him to take it so hard. Through his sobs, he announced he would move into Grandma and Grandpa's house until it grew back. "Why would you want to do that?" I asked. His answer was "I'm afraid you are going to look scary." I was afraid of looking scary too. We talked for a long while and I was able to reassure him that I would still look like his Mom. I told him about my wig. In hindsight, it would have been helpful to have it on hand (it was on order) when I had the initial discussion with him.

About a week before my long hair was due to fall out, I cut it short. Fearful that I would fall apart at the salon, I asked my hairdresser to come to the house. My husband took the boys out for dinner. I opened a bottle of wine and in the time it takes to drink a glass of pinot noir I had a hairdo to match my new profession, soldier/warrior. That evening may have been tougher for my hairdresser than it was for me. She was young and had never dealt with a situation quite like that. I think I held it together for her. She left refusing to accept any money.

Even with my new short "do", I couldn't imagine how my hair was just going to fall out. Sure my scalp felt weird at times but every time I gave my hair a little tug it was met with resistance. Then one day my little tug yielded a pinch of hair. I didn't even feel it coming out. It was time. I returned to the wig shop where my girlfriend and I had been the week before. My new "hairdresser" was expecting me. She had done this before, way too many times according to her. We went into a private room and when I came out my new wig fit snuggly on head. Eventually, almost all the hair on my body would disappear, even my eyelashes. Apparently, women have eyelashes for a reason not related to mascara. It seems as though they are there to keep stuff out of our eyes. It's amazing how much dust and debris finds its way into your eye when your lashes aren't there to protect them. In a cruel twist, the hair for which I had no use hung on when all the others had gone. I speak of my leg hair which continued to grow as if to mock me in a spiteful way.

I was never really comfortable in a wig. The radio and television coverage about my cancer evoked a lot of good will and a lot of questions too. It seemed as though everyone in south Florida knew I was going through chemotherapy. Some would inquire as to why my hair had not fallen out. Others would remark that I didn't look like a cancer patient. Inevitably it always came back to the hair. I remember one afternoon when my husband and I attended the NASCAR championship. My counts were up and I would be around thousands of people. The potential for well meaning but insensitive questions was huge. I chose to wear a scarf that day to circumvent all the hair questions. I thought to myself, you want to know what a cancer patient looks like, well here I am, and yes my hair fell out.

More difficult than the questions from strangers was the fact that I was unrecognizable to people who had known me for years. One afternoon at my son's school, a woman walked up to me and introduced herself. The problem was that I had known her for quite a while. We had been out to dinner together and I had even been to her house. I was devastated. I cried for days. But I took something away from that experience. I realized that we (people) in general don't really look into one another's eyes. We're too busy looking at the hair and figure, the jewelry and clothing. I vowed to not be so distracted by all the trappings of modern day primping and to look at a persons face. Faces are beautiful!

All told, I bought four wigs and enough bandanas and scarves to fill a dresser drawer. Oh yes, and lots of hats too. Wigs allow for experimentation with different hair styles and colors. My husband liked the red one. I recommend buying at least one wig that matches your real hair color because as your hair starts to grow back, it can be seen around the hairline. Wigs require very little care and cut down on the time spent getting ready to go out. They also hold up really well in humid climates. Unfortunately, I hated the way the wig felt on my head. Besides, it's hard to wear sunglasses with a wig. I kept a baseball cap in the car for the times when I couldn't wait to get home before ripping it off my head. I went with bandanas and scarves most of the time. I found that look to be a guy repellent which was OK with me at the time.

As my hair grew back, it came in unruly and difficult to manage. Urged on by my partner in crime Jackie, I got a full head of hair extensions. I didn't know how happy they would make me, but wow, having nice hair again really helped me move on. Hair extensions are very costly, however, and it can be hard to find a hairdresser who is experienced enough to handle the challenge. Once I had them though, I had to answer a whole new set of questions like, "how did your hair grow back so fast?' I really didn't mind though, hey if celebrities can get extension for no reason, why not me?

After two sets of hair extensions, I was comfortable with the length of my hair. It was still hard to manage because the chemotherapy had changed its texture. My hairdresser suggested I use a Brazilian hair straightening product on it. The product did not damage my hair and it felt smooth again. I couldn't have been happier with my new "do".

TAMARA

I have to admit that I was mortified at the thought of losing my hair. I had been growing it long for years, spent numerous hours and tons of money. It was my pride and joy.

My biggest fear when I found out I had breast cancer was whether or not I would need chemotherapy. "Will I lose my hair?" loomed in the back of my mind. I was able to keep it together; in fact I was fairly calm in all my doctors' appointments until I asked my breast surgeon, "Do you think I will need chemotherapy?" When she said yes, I broke down and cried like a baby. She said, "It's always the hair that gets them crying, never mind the major surgery."

Once I had accepted I would lose my hair, I decided to donate it to Locks of Love an organization that makes wigs for children with cancer or other diseases that make them lose their hair.

I was told my hair would start to fall out about 14 days after my first chemotherapy treatment. Sure enough, I woke up one morning with the weirdest feeling like the back of my hair was all standing up on end, but when I reached back it wasn't. My head began to tingle and itch and some strands started to come out in my hand and brush. I went the next day to get it shaved off. I didn't cry, but my husband almost did. He threatened to shave his own head too, but I wouldn't let him. It didn't hit me until a few days later when my husband suggested that we run to the store. I totally panicked; I thought I couldn't go anywhere. I don't have any hair! I broke down and sobbed, I felt I would never get up the nerve to leave the house.

It wasn't until I saw my sister, who was also bald from chemotherapy, that I felt better. If she could do it, then so could I. I quickly got used to it. I would throw on a hat, bandana or my wig and just go.

As chemotherapy progressed, there did come a point where my lack of hair didn't bother me as much. I was weak and tired and simply didn't have the energy to be concerned as much about it. The upside was at least I didn't have to take care of my hair when I felt so bad.

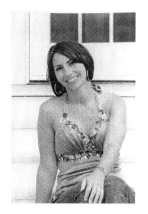
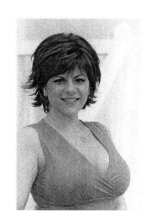

HELPFUL TIPS FOR FEELING GOOD
MAKEUP

Treat yourself to a free makeover at a cosmetic counter

EYES

Cargo, eyeliner (cream and powder set)

EYEBROWS

Begin filling in your eyebrows before you lose them, the extra practice is helpful
MAC Powder
Anastasia of Beverly Hills (Eyebrow Set)

EYELASHES

False eyelashes

WIG

Try on wigs prior to losing your hair.
Synthetic wigs are easier to maintain.
Wig/Mastectomy Stores usually carry "hats with hair". These are baseball hats
with hair attachments.

CLOTHING

Pajama tops and shirts with buttons or zippers are most comfortable after breast surgery.

"It's Hard to Wear Sunglasses, With a Wig,"

—Gina

GINA

Maintaining a positive self image can be challenging for a woman going through breast cancer treatment, but with a little creativity and a positive outlook, her beauty shines right through. Boca Raton Community Hospital, where I received my treatments, is conveniently located near a fabulous mall. So before I began chemotherapy, between scans and doctors appointments, I would often wonder through trying to forget my misery. I used the time to pick up a few essential products and many non essential self-pity items as well. My husband, God love him, would say "go buy yourself something, you deserve it." On the days I was medicated, my American Express would see a lot of action. It all worked out though, because my purchases came in handy when I no longer felt like going out.

I was told that chemotherapy gives you really clear skin. I found this to be true! My skin tone changed a little too and at times it was sallow. Fortunately, during one of my pity retail therapy sessions, I purchased cosmetics. Since my immune system was going to be weak, I decided to purge my makeup stash. I replaced the old stuff with fresh new products. I got some neutral blush and some creamy eye shadow. I also purchased several new eyeliner pencils and some eyebrow powder and a brush. These helped me to avoid the washed out look as my eyelashes and brows became thin. I even threw caution to the wind and grabbed a few pairs of false eyelashes for special occasions.

I used gentle cleansers on my skin followed by great smelling body lotions containing natural ingredients. Minty foot creams for my sore feet were also a nice treat. Facials helped me keep a "healthy" glow on my face.

Although my wardrobe became a collection of hoodies and jeans, I occasionally dressed up and went somewhere other than a doctor's office. My husband and I basically shut down our social calendar. We chose our events carefully, most often involving a charity. I shopped on line a little, choosing blousy tops or jackets. Taking a few pairs of pants to the tailor for alterations proved to be a good idea. They fit my slimmer chemotherapy body better and helped me to avoid looking sickly. And for the finishing touch, I wore my jewelry, more often than before. After all, what was I saving it for? Everyday was special.

Shoe shopping became extremely gratifying. No matter what was happening up top, my feet remained the same size. At times while I was waiting in a doctor's office, staring at the floor, I would catch a glimpse of my fabulous shoes and smile. Several months after my chemotherapy began, I suffered from a lot of foot pain. I chose to wear more comfortable shoes. Yet another reason to buy shoes—flats.

Underneath my façade, I had an ever changing chest. At first I was swollen on one side with a tumor, and then I was disfigured by a mastectomy. Afterward, the tissue expanders gave sort of a bad boob job look, too high and hard. Then there was the deflation for radiation which left me slightly lop sided. I compensated accordingly with a variety of bras, sports bras, tank bras and loose shirts. At times I wore little silicone bra inserts nicknamed "Chicken cutlets" by my girlfriend. They cost about $35.00 a pair and can be purchased at many lingerie stores or departments. Other times I wore real prosthesis fitted by a professional at Nordstrom. These cost over $200.00 each! Some insurance companies will pay for them with the proper paperwork. Happily, things look good at the top these days. After five surgeries, it's back to the beach.

I mention exercise last because I didn't do a lot of it. I was on my way to the gym on the day I was diagnosed and I haven't been back since. Sadly, I sort of fell out, focusing what was left of my energy on my family. Just being there to participate in family life was exhausting. When I felt good, a gentle yoga class or a walk was the activity of choice. Happily; my desire to exercise has returned and I love to practice Bikram yoga several times a week, walk, swim and play with my boys.

TAMARA

As a Veterinarian, it was easier for me to wear a bandana to work everyday. I had one in every color. My wigs would become itchy and hot during the day. I chose instead to wear them when I went out with family and friends. It made me feel normal again.

Today's wigs are very realistic. I ended up with four different ones. I had different lengths and different colors. I had fun changing my look. However, I strongly recommend your first wig to be similar to your real hair. This will help you feel more like yourself.

I always wondered what people would do if one day when it was raining, I just whipped off my wig and ran to the car bald. The thought always made me laugh, but I never did it. I did go bald on South Beach in Miami one day. I have to say, I think I fit right in!

CINDY

Prior to my surgery, I decided to cut my below-shoulder-length hair to a bob slightly below my chin. I knew I would need time to adjust to losing my hair. I figured I would cut my hair in stages migrating to a pixie cut during chemotherapy until it was time to shave it.

I don't know why, but during this time I seemed to be assaulted with images of bald women/girls. The local newspaper had a picture of a teenager shaving her head for a fundraiser at her high school on the front page. Even with tears in her eyes, she held her arms up in victory for the very noble cause of raising money for Cancer research. The reality T.V. show American Inventor showed a woman with Alopecia. She bared her bald head to help market her invention (an absorbent pad to be used with wigs, hats, helmets etc.).

It was strange. Before, I had lived a relatively Cancer-free existence. Almost overnight my life changed and I saw Cancer, and specifically Breast Cancer everywhere in the media.

I had my wigs selected and my baseball hat with hair attachment and 20 colored bandanas ordered and ready to go weeks before actually needing them.

On day 19 after chemotherapy started, my friend (who had supported her mother as she fought breast Cancer the year prior) came over with a buzzer in hand and shaved my head. No, I didn't feel triumphant like Demi Moore in GI Jane. I was more in shock, a little numb and still not 100% sure this wasn't a dream.

I started wearing my wigs. They seemed to have their own identity so I named the long ones Tiffany One and Two and the short one Maxine. Friends and family were supportive of my new looks. The best thing about wigs is that they always look good. You can whip them off in a moment's notice. You can get caught in a rainstorm and look better than most people!

I can't lie. I was never comfortable enough to go bald in public. I didn't want to wear scarves. I didn't like the way I looked or felt in them. I felt they screamed "Bald Cancer Patient!" However, the moment I got home, off came the wig. My family and closest friends saw the bald me and always made me feel good about myself. I can't say I ever felt like a sexy, hot bald woman, but I was damn close a couple of times.

The moment I finished chemotherapy I started watching for any signs of regrowth. I took a multi vitamin specifically designed to help hair grow. I watched as I went from bald, bald, bald, a little shadow, a lot of shadow, pricklies, fuzzy chicken to pixie. Now, a year and a half later my wavy hair has come back downright curly ala a dark haired Shirley Temple.

HELPFUL RESOURCES AND BOOKS

WEBSITES:

www.y-me.com
www.breastrecon.com
www.komen.org
www.breastcancer.org
www.youngsurvival.org
www.cancer.org
www.save2ndbase.com

BOOKS:

The Breast Reconstruction Guidebook
By Kathy Steligo
101—Questions and Answers About Breast Cancer
by Zora K. Brown
Waking the Warrior Goddess: Dr. Christine Horner's Program to Protect Against & Fight Breast Cancer
by Christine Horner
After Breast Cancer: A Common-Sense Guide to Life After Treatment
by Hester Schnipper, LICSW
Breast Cancer Husband: How to Help Your Wife (and Yourself) during Diagnosis, Treatment and Beyond
by Marc Silver

FOR CHILDREN:

Metu and Lee Learn about Breast Cancer by Dr. Shenin Sachedina
The Chemo Cat by Cathy Nilson

Being upset about losing your hair is okay. It's more than okay. It is normal. Although at this time, losing your hair due to breast cancer chemotherapy is a reality, it doesn't mean you can't be upset about it. It can be distressing and depressing.

Long after the chemotherapy is done there will still be very little hair. But as it grows back and your eyebrows and eyelashes return, pictures of health and wellness become your reflections in the mirror.

CHAPTER SIX

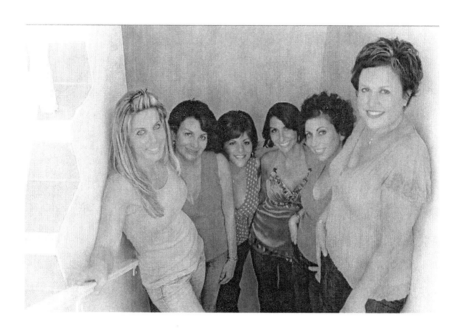

SUPPORT:
THE SISTERHOOD

"What helped me the most was my support group. These women had walked in my shoes, and they knew the path I was walking on."

—Donna

The support section of our book is especially important for caregivers as well as survivors. It offers a vision of what each of us deemed as important and meaningful in the way of support. As you read this chapter, be mindful of the loved one you are trying to help, even if that someone is you. There are many ways to give support and many ways to find it. Whether you are experiencing this journey yourself or with someone, you are not alone.

The second part of this chapter is written by our support systems. They were our loved ones who lived through the day to day battles with us. There are stories from our young children, teenagers, husbands, significant others, parents and friends. The chapter also contains the profound and often surprising ways our cancer diagnoses affected the people around us. Read on as we share our secrets of strength that made it possible for us to persevere.

DONNA

Support has overflowed from family and friends and sometimes even from strangers! The support that helped me the most came from my involvement in our support group. It was so beneficial that all these women had walked in my shoes and they knew the path that I was walking on. It has been a great tool to share problems, questions, concerns, feeling and experiences. The support group has also been a great way to meet a lot of awesome ladies! This was not the way that I would have wanted to meet these women but, to be honest, probably would have never met them if not for breast cancer. Just another perk of having breast cancer! The bond that we all share will last a lifetime. We will all remember the warmth, caring and support we received from each other and we'll say, "Oh yea, I remember I had breast cancer twenty-five years ago!" The support group has been the "silver lining" on the entire cancer experience.

I remember the first time I walked into the support group meeting room. I thought to myself "Oh my God, where did all these young girls come from with breast cancer!?" I guess I was expecting a room full of older ladies. In one way, I thought it was tragic for so many young women to be in this situation and also pleasantly surprised and relieved to meet people I could relate to on so many levels. I have always been the type of person to get involved, and I was open to discussing my experience with breast cancer. I would highly recommend someone who isn't as open or out going as me, to step-out and try a support group. Give it a shot, if you don't like one, try another, seek until you find. I don't see how someone can go over this hurdle of breast cancer without a support group.

What helped lift my spirits the most was knowing that people were praying for me. The outpouring of caring and concern was comforting. Friends and family called on a regular basis to check-up on me show that they cared. They also helped lift my spirits with their positive energy and thoughts. All of my doctor's showed they cared by listening to me and not making me feel like just a number.

Nice cards and gifts came from so many thoughtful people. It was so amazing that people I really didn't know well reached out to me. It was overwhelming at times, the kindness of strangers. I recall a young lady that was sitting at a table adjacent to me at Einstein's restaurant. She could see that I was reading an article about breast cancer that my eyes were tearing up. She got up out of her chair, came up to me and gave me a side hug and said some nice things. That courageous stranger gave me just what I needed at that moment. Several family members sent me money to help with hospital bills. My parents would drive down from Orlando at the drop of a hat to help and spend time with me. Cindy and

Tomi from my support group spent New Years Eve with me in a hospital emergency room. We watched the ball come down together. Happy New Year! I sure wasn't feeling it at that moment but I knew better times were coming.

My chemotherapy nurses were always in a good mood and positive. They always treated me with care and concern. My girlfriends were always there to lend a hand, be my cheerleaders, encourage me and lend support. All the girls in my support group have been a Godsend, I can't say enough about them. My brothers and sister would call to check up on a regular basis and offered me financial support if I needed it. My best friend Patrick would call me everyday to check up on me. He brought me food on several occasions. Most of all, he was my emotional support. He was the one that put up with me when I was sad, scared, or just feeling crappy. He was also my biggest supporter. I am very grateful to have had him on my side. ALL THESE PEOPLE WERE MY ANGELS!!

DEBBIE

Dealing with a serious illness not only affects you, but so many others around you. My greatest source of strength and support came from my family. They exhibited the true meaning of team work. Each one in their own way helped me and helped each other.

People are often saying how proud they are of me. Yet, what immediately comes to mind is how proud I am of my family. I stand a little taller when I think of my husband getting the kids ready for school before work. Then, he would return home after a long day, just in time to give the kids a bath so that they could "look handsome" for mommy as they gave their goodnight kisses. Then, he would take the few free hours left in his day to spend with me, comfort me, tell me how beautiful I am and how much he loves me.

I smile a little wider when I think of my then four and six year old boys, their never ending kisses and hugs, even when I had little energy and no hair. Their unconditional love and genuine spirits gave me the courage I needed to endure this journey.

I feel more secure when I think of my parents and in-laws who filled in where ever they were needed without question and without being asked. They got done whatever needed to get done to make sure we, as a family, moved forward everyday.

Whoever gives you strength and support during this difficult time, embrace it. Hold on to the lessons you will learn about the true character of people. This more than anything is what has changed me the most throughout my journey. I only hope I can live up the great examples of human compassion that was shown to me and hopefully become a better person because of it.

TAMARA

I found support through many different avenues. My husband was my biggest supporter. My family and friends were wonderful. I joined a support group and had an older sister who was literally just a few months ahead of me on her journey battling breast cancer.

On a daily basis, my husband, Tim, took care of me. It amazes me, even today when I think about the day we learned that I had breast cancer. It was only three short months after our wedding. He is such a strong and loving man. I feel that very few men would have made it through this journey, especially since we had only been a part of each others lives for such a relatively short time. It is a credit to his character, knowing that he didn't sign up for this when we got married, yet he never made me feel that this wasn't part of "the plan".

My friends helped more than I could have ever imagined. One woman named Gwen, whom I met through my husband three years ago, was a huge inspiration for me. The manner in which she deals with life and her own health issues is admirable. We spent many a nights sitting and discussing our myriad of health problems. She was always there for me. She may not realize it, but she was a bright light for me in some of my darkest hours.

I have also made friendships through my support group that I know will last a lifetime. I felt a sudden deep sense of calm and attachment to these women. No one else knows quite what breast cancers like unless, especially emotionally, they have experienced it. Even my husband, who saw me go through it all, did not understand completely. I felt something very satisfying in my soul, knowing that someone else knew exactly how I felt. My support group gave me comfort and peace when I could not find it anywhere else.

My parents and my sister provided their own unique kind of support. My mom and dad, who were already actively immersed in my sister's battle when I was diagnosed, were invaluable to me. I drew strength from them daily. Something else that was of enormous strength to me during my battle with breast cancer was my sister. I had always looked up to her and now more than ever, her strength and grace carried me through. Although, I was filled with such sadness that she, too, was going through this, I was also selfishly glad to have had her go through this with me. We have always had a special bond, but we have gotten even closer through our journey. I always knew, no matter how scared or sick I was, I could call her and feel better. If she could do it, so could I!

Even though the battle is over, the war is still ongoing. I know that there will be good times and bad times. I will be forever thankful for my husband, my parents, my sister and friends.

GINA

The body cannot heal if there is a disease in the mind. I found my sanity through my support group. It was then that I was able to reclaim my health. I first met Jackie when the nurse at our plastic surgeon's office asked me if she could pass on my name to a new patient who needed to talk. I agreed, but commented that I wasn't that strong myself. I was in the midst of chemotherapy and a mastectomy; she had yet to begin. What could I possibly say to help her, knowing the hell that was to come? The first time we connected, we spent 40 minutes on the phone. She helped me as much as I helped her.

We agreed to meet at the hospital's monthly support group. I would wear my wig (really a scarf gal) so Jackie could see how it looked. The feeling in the room was one of acceptance. It was warm and comfortable. The life flame in each of us seemed to burn a little brighter. We were stronger together. So began a sisterhood that I treasure. There were at least ten of us in the room that night, including the some of the authors of this book. Afterward we went to dinner and talked for hours. Boy did our waiter get an earful, poor guy! There was even a show and tell in the ladies' room. Even now we still meet monthly to share and support. We do it for ourselves.

Having gone through six months of treatment before I found these wonderful women, my suggestion for newly diagnosed women would be to find a group. Do it soon. Check with your treatment facility or through local organizations like the American Cancer Society. If the first group you try doesn't fit, try another. Most of the girls agree that their families encourage them to go, even if it means eating take out that night. Many of our husband's have noticed that we seem happier when we get home from a night out. I often hire a baby sitter for the evening to help my son with his homework. For those that can't get a sitter, this is a good time to take some one up on one of those "If there's anything I can do" offers. If you just can't make it to a group, reach out on the internet.

The new friendships I've developed since I began this fight are such a gift. I was one of those girls who was more like one the guys, many of my close friends are men. But now I have a whole new group of girlfriends for whom I will always be grateful. We are each unique but we are the same. We have been through the initiation and now belong to a club no one wants to join. I look forward to the day when we have no new members.

Prior to my diagnosis, my family had little experience in dealing with cancer. We were a lucky bunch, happily taking our lives for granted. When I first became sick and the horror of my disease began to sink in, my husband Paul became my rock. Along with the fear of dying, I was afraid of what the chemotherapy and the mastectomy would do to my physical appearance. Realizing how fragile my psyche had become, he constantly reassured me how much our life together meant to him. He would tell me "all I want is your head on a plate." His love was unconditional.

During my treatment, he became a phone screener, internet researcher, meal coordinator, and car pool driver, a regular Mr. Mom/Super Dad combined. Paul insisted we get a housekeeper, because he didn't want me to waste the moments when I was feeling good on housework. He sent regular email updates to all our family and friends. He put up with my mood swings and petty jealousies even when I was sure other women where waiting for me to die so they could have a chance with him. Through everything, he managed to look at the sweaty hairless creature (me) lying next to him in bed with love in his eyes. When I was really down he would say "head on a plate," and we would smile.

Not only did he put on a brave face for me, but for his radio listening audience as well. It was quite difficult for him to go to work day after day pretending everything was great, laughing at silly things and entertaining the masses. So, together we decided that is would be best to let everyone know what was going on. With his buddies from the show by his side, he announced to the South Florida radio audience that I was ill. Just like that, hundreds of thousands of people knew that I fighting breast cancer. The phone began to ring and hundreds of touching emails and cards poured in, some folks wrote that they had to pull over on the highway when they heard the news because they were crying. The UPS guy arrived at my door everyday with gifts and remedies, supplements and books—too many to count. The community had embraced us, and we were humbled.

Through it all my husband remained strong; he became the face of breast cancer husbands. I know it was hard for him to answer questions about me everywhere he went. Surely, he would've rather been talking about fishing. He embraced my new friends and participated in cancer walks. He helped raise money for research too. He honored our marriage vow of: in sickness and in health with reverence.

From the moment of my diagnosis, my two children inspired me to get well. I remember telling the nurse who was with me at the time, "I can't die, I have two boys at home who need me." When the fear of the chemotherapy and the surgery began to overwhelm me, I would focus on them. In my darkest sickest hours, it was the thought of leaving them to be raised by someone else that kept me in the fight. I got sick in early September, the start of the school year and what a year it was going to be. AJ was starting kindergarten at a brand new school and the Nic was beginning his eighth grade year at the same Catholic school I attended as a child. As we braced ourselves for the unknown, one thing was certain, there would be a lot of hand washing going on at my house.

My youngest, AJ, was five. It's hard to know just how he processed the information we told him about my illness. On the most basic level, he didn't even want to share a bag of chips with me because he was afraid of the cancer germs. We had to explain to him that you can't catch cancer. AJ grew tired of having his mom always going to the doctor and being too sick to play. There was a constant flow of babysitters and housekeepers, more than ever before. He was bothered by my hair loss. Eventually, though, he told me that he was getting used to my new look, I was the same Mom just without hair. Ah, if only that were true. I tried my best to stay involved with his new school and routine. I remember one evening when I was helping him with his homework. He was writing a sentence and asked me how to spell the word 'were'. I could not do it. My chemo brain was so bad at that moment that the letters would not come to me. I had to get out the dictionary. When we finished, I was sure that the cancer had gone to my brain. How could I be so dumb? I owe a debt of gratitude to my son's teachers who loved on him a little more and demanded a little less. When permission slips and projects were late, they would send home gentle reminders—never making him feel different or out of sync with the rest of the class. Things got better, but as my Herceptin treatments intruded on our summer vacation and then into his first grade year, it was clear that my whole family was growing weary. He wanted it to be over so badly that even today, I sometimes hide the fact that I'm going to the doctor so he won't become anxious that I might be sick again. Through it all, however, he remained a love who would cuddle with me after school and ask me how I was feeling. Until recently I hadn't realized just how affected he was by all the drama, but then in a moment that broke my heart, all the awfulness of my disease reared its' ugly head. AJ had a stomach virus, he was vomiting violently and his tummy hurt. He was lying on the couch writhing in pain and cried out "I hope I don't have cancer." Wow, I thought. The fear has crept into his mind and stolen part of his innocence.

My older son Nic seemed less disturbed by all the turmoil. He was having a big year at school. His routine remained fairly consistent. When I asked him about how he felt when I got sick, he said "I didn't want to believe it. I didn't want to believe you could die." Perhaps that's why he didn't really acknowledge the problem very often. A typical teenager, he was the center of his universe and that was OK. His teachers were also especially kind to him. Many of the teachers and Nuns at his school also taught me when I was a student there. Because we had been a part of the school community for so many years, it was easier for the other Moms to rally around us. They drove carpool and brought meals. I would get loving phone messages reminding me of important dates not to be missed during that all important eighth grade year. The ladies even organized a Christmas tree decorating party to help me decorate our thirteen foot tree. It took six ladies four hours and when it was over, my tree had never looked better. They even held a beautiful prayer service for me the night before my mastectomy. For me it was an affirmation of love. For Nic, it was a year complete with a high school entrance exam and grad night at Disney World. He didn't miss a thing. Mission accomplished.

I consider my lifelong friends to be one of the great blessings in my life, many of whom I've known since childhood. Through it all, my friends were there—close when I needed them, at a distance when I needed space. They delivered meals 5 nights a week for months. Everyone got together and threw me a birthday party. My husband made sure it wasn't a surprise party though because that could have backfired. I would need to rest up and prepare to celebrate. They sent cards and gifts and took me to lunch when I was up to it. Some of the guys even organized a football weekend and insisted I come. (I love football) When I told them that my Herceptin treatment might leave me feeling too sick to attend the game, they assured me it would be no problem, telling me if I needed to leave the game early, we'd all leave together. "We can hang out in the hotel if you want just as long as we are together," they told me. I was so touched by all the phone calls, but more so when one of the guys would call. It must have been so uncomfortable to ask about breast cancer, I'm sure they struggled with what they would say, but they did it and I will always be grateful.

I truly believe my friends and family willed me to get better. I am so glad I reached out to them. Since that time, one of the women from my son's school has been diagnosed. She also reached out and many loving hands were there to help.

JACKIE

I had a tremendous amount of support from my family, friends and neighbors. I felt so lucky, yet it was kind of a double edged sword. As much as I appreciated everyone's concern for me, all I really wanted was to be with my husband, my kids or other women that were going through what I was going through. I felt like nobody knew what to say to me and I didn't really know what to say to them. I didn't want people feeling sorry for me. I knew I was going to get through this; I just wanted to focus all my energy on fighting the cancer and finishing my treatment.

I joined a support group that was suggested to me by my doctors. I felt an instant connection and sense of belonging to virtual strangers. As bizarre as the idea of this sounds, this diverse group of women have ended up becoming my good friends that I know will always be a part of my life.

I am so appreciative of my supportive and devoted husband after 21 years of marriage. I am very grateful for my three beautiful and courageous children that stayed strong and gave me the will to beat this. I am forever thankful for the insight and strength that my new found "cancer sisters" have given.

CINDY

About ten days before my mastectomy, I felt ready to find a support group where I could connect with others who were going through this similar experience. The social worker from the multi-modality clinic suggested a young women's breast cancer networking group. This group appealed to me because it was geared towards women under 50 who had been diagnosed within the last year.

I remember walking into the meeting room and being the first one there. I sat there with my jeweled journal and a list of possible questions for the other women IF I got up the nerve to speak.

A young woman came in a few minutes later. I was struck by how pretty she was. Later, I would come to learn this was Tamara. We said "Hello" and then just sat there waiting for others to arrive. As the time passed others entered until there were about eight of us in the room. I looked at each woman and wondered what her story was. "Was she wearing a wig? Did she have a mastectomy?" I felt overwhelmed. We sat around a square table and the social worker facilitated the meeting. We started by going around the room introducing ourselves and telling our individual "stories." Each person was at a different stage in their journey. Some were almost one year out from their diagnosis date. Some were in the middle of chemotherapy. There I was, the only person who hadn't had surgery yet. When I told my story, I remember feeling instant understanding and compassion from these strangers who instantly felt like close friends.

After the meeting, Jackie, Gina, Tamara and I decided to go get something to eat and continue talking. Little did I know these three women would become my instant family—my cancer sisters. With each upcoming event and milestone, these incredible women would be there for me, share with me and allow me to participate in their incredible journey.

As the months passed, the group would slowly evolve. The "Seniors"—women who were at least one year out—would slowly leave the group and newly diagnosed women would join. I was always so sad to see a new woman enter the group, sad that another young woman would have to go through what I had gone through. But I was glad to know that we could be there for her to help her as others had helped me.

Throughout my journey I was amazed how family, friends and strangers rallied to love and support me. To keep everybody updated I started a blog on a free blog website. This was a great way for me journal my feelings and still keep everybody updated without telling the same story over and over again.

To this day, I am amazed by the secret angels who appeared to offer a word of kindness, give a gift of arm pillows and a blanket, and help me lift or carry something without having to "tell my story."

I will forever be grateful to those who participated in my journey—those who are still in my life and those who I believe were brought into to my life for the sole purpose of supporting me.

CAREGIVERS: WELCOME TO THE CLUB

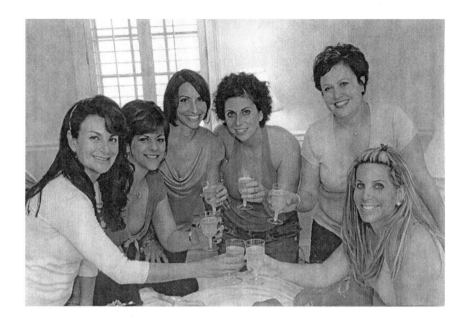

ETHAN (age 5), DEBBIE'S SON

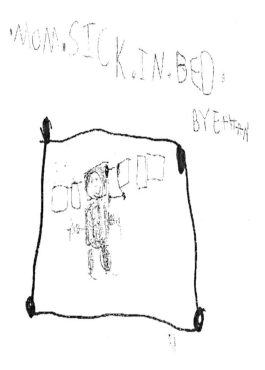

ISAAC (age 7), DEBBIE'S SON

When my mom first told my little brother, Ethan, and I she was sick, I was a little worried. She said that she was going to have to take some very yucky medicine that would make her tired and probably have to rest in bed a lot. She also said that the medicine was going to make her hair fall out but it would grow back. I told her she should just wear a wig or a bandana. My little brother didn't really believe that her hair would fall out. I didn't really care. It didn't bother me.

When my mom started taking the yucky medicine I started getting worried and scared. I was afraid that my mom might die. Even though no one likes to take medicine, my mom took all of her medicine. She had to take the medicine eight times. If you take all of your medicine and believe in yourself, you will be ok. I know my mom believed in herself and that she would be ok.

I was so happy after she took her medicine for the eighth time. I was glad when she was done taking her medicine. She really was getting better and her hair was growing back.

I love my mom with short hair. I think she looks really cute like that. Most of all, I just love my mom!

DEBBIE'S FRIEND, LEE

Growing up, my parents instilled many values in me. They taught me right from wrong. They taught me to have manners and to be kind to others. They taught me to love unconditionally and fully. They prepared me to work hard to overcome obstacles that might come my way. Still, there was one thing that all of these life lessons never taught me. What to say or do when your dear friend tells you that she has breast cancer. When I was young, I remember hearing about "cancer" (in a whisper) but never really new what it meant, never new the depths of how it affects your body, your mind, and your spirit. I had absolutely no idea how this experience would not only change my friend's life, as well as the lives of her family members, but would also change my life as well.

When Debbie first told me she had found a lump in her breast and was going to have the lump removed I knew it was nothing. I knew it was just going to be a cyst or something benign and that she would be fine in a day or two. It wasn't. In fact, it was far worse than I ever could have imagined. It was much worse than Debbie and her family could have imagined either. She eventually found out that she had Stage II breast cancer and that it had spread to seven of her lymph nodes. She was going to have to have a port put into her chest, 8 sessions of chemotherapy and 6 weeks of radiation treatment after that. This was absolutely implausible, just beyond comprehension. How could this happen to someone so vibrant, young and healthy? This was just devastating.

What is amazing about my friend Debbie is that she approaches everything in her life with a sense of calmness, a sense of "put—togetherness" and a true sense of ease. Also gently infused into this lovely life fluidity is her ability to always laugh, smile, and love life to the absolute fullest, whether it be celebrating the milestone of a birthday or anniversary, or something as small as her child's first loose tooth. It might sound cliché, but if you could look up the definition of "zest for life" in the dictionary, you would surely find her picture there! If there is one thing that actually defines Debbie though, I would have to say that it is her devotion to her family. She is the quintessential mother hen, nurturing, protecting, and loving her family. If anyone could fight this tough fight, I knew it would be her. She loves nothing more in this world than her family, and I knew that there was a warrior deep inside her that she would summons, just so that she would be ok, for the sake of her family.

She approached her cancer diagnosis the exact same way that she approaches life, which meant that she would do everything in her power to get through this, all the while doing so with positive attitude, strong character and a keen mind. She made it her mission to learn everything she possibly could about her cancer in a calm, yet aggressive and intelligent manner. She obtained all the information she could, she commissioned the best doctors she could, and she prepared herself to process, organize and attack. With her amazing husband and supportive family and friends behind her, I knew that she was in the best hands possible, that she would battle her cancer with a vengeance, and that she would ultimately triumph.

Debbie and I spoke on the phone several times a day throughout this entire journey. I was desperate to know everything, I wanted to be there for her in any and every way possible, to support her, to understand what she was about to go through. In order to do so, I needed an education too. I was thankful that even through her own personal nightmare, she had the patience to take the time to help me understand the medical treatment that she was receiving, and what "the plan" was going to be. This enabled me to ask the right questions after each step and enabled me to know what to expect, like how she would feel, what she would need, and what's next on this rocky path ahead of us.

So now I was armed with an incredible amount of new knowledge, and I felt competent to talk to her and her family about all of the medical steps that she would be facing. However, I was still left with a hollowing and unanswered question. What could I actually DO to help her? What could I really DO to help make this better for her, if that was even possible? If I could just snap my fingers and make this all go away, I would have, but obviously, I could not. However, there was one thing that I knew would make her feel somewhat peaceful and calm, and perhaps relieved throughout this ordeal. It was for her to know that her family, the single most important thing to her, was ok, was comfortable, and was as happy as possible, considering the circumstances. So I instinctually went full speed ahead doing something that I thankfully knew I could do. Love my friend and her family unconditionally and fully. There were pickups after school and lots of play dates at my house with her boys. There were playing silly games and lots of hugs and tickles. There was also the occasional discussion with her boys about how strong and amazing their Mom is, and the subtle and gentle encouragement about how she was going to be just fine. Hopefully the occasional brisket and potatoes didn't hurt either; perhaps some "comfort food" would add a little comfort to this amazingly dynamic family that somehow managed to keep it all together. I still didn't think this was enough, but it was the very least I could do.

Maybe it was comforting or helpful for Debbie in some way to talk and to discuss things with someone who wasn't actively involved in making the medical decisions for her and with her. Whatever the reason, I felt lucky and grateful that she let me "in". I'm grateful Debbie allowed me to encourage her to go outside on little outings throughout her treatment, as difficult as it was for her to face the world. I'm glad I was able to be there for her and tell her how pretty her "new hair" (her wig) looked, as it was truly perfect every single day! I'm grateful she let me know how sick she actually felt on some days so I could try to help comfort her with something so simple as a cool iced tea, soothing words, or just a big hug and an old-fashioned "good cry". She knew what was right for her and she was a champ at letting those around her know, without saying a word, what she needed both physically and emotionally.

I still don't think Debbie has any idea about how her fight to beat breast cancer has affected so many people around her. The way she handled herself during the darkest of days has changed the way I view obstacles, people and life. She fought her cancer so valiantly and so nobly. Just knowing Debbie and being by her side during all of this has made me feel lucky to have a friend who is brave and strong, and so real and genuine in all facets of her life. She has made me appreciate every single minute we are all blessed to be on this earth surrounded by our loved ones and enjoying the precious moments that make up the memories of our lives. She is an inspiration to her children, her husband, her family, her friends, and actually, all who know her. She is the ultimate example of how to handle and overcome the most frightening of situations with gritty persistence, unwavering integrity and most of all, true grace. I know that Debbie did not like how she looked without any hair. However, standing in the bathroom with her that day as we shaved her head, I thought she never looked more beautiful, as to me, it was her badge of honor, courage, and hope. She is a true hero in my book.

MICHELLE (age 14), JACKIE'S DAUGHTER

The day I found out my mom had breast cancer is a day I will never forget. My brother had just picked me up from dinner. As soon as I got in the car he said, "No matter what Mom tells you, don't cry!"

When we got home, I headed straight for my mom's room. She was sitting on her bed with the mother of one of my friends who was a breast cancer survivor. Unable to stop myself, I began crying. I knew at that second my mom had breast cancer.

Whenever I would talk about my mom's breast cancer, everyone kept telling me to stay strong, and everything would be ok. That is easier said than done. I tried, but I kept thinking in my head, will I grow up without my mom?"

Something else that was difficult for me was my mom's hair loss. Growing up, people were always commenting on how amazing my mom's hair was. My mom always had long hair and she always looked beautiful. The day she lost her hair was not easy for my family. We felt awful for her. It was especially hard for me, as her daughter, to deal with the idea that she was had no hair and was going to wear a wig. It just seemed so crazy. It didn't seem real.

It was real, though, and my family was dealing with her cancer everyday. My mom wore her wig everywhere. I have to say, it may not have been her real hair, but it sure did the trick! I really don't think anyone knew it was a wig, unless she told them. Still, I know it was upsetting for her and that was hard. Finally, when my mom's hair started growing back, everyday she asked me, "Is my hair getting longer?" The only answer (for my mom's sake) was yes. But, yes, was the true answer. Something I have learned from this experience is that hair is just hair and it grows back. Just give it time.

Another thing I learned is how to be strong and brave. Seeing someone you love go through something as hard as breast cancer treatment is tough. It takes a lot of courage. She was strong for herself and for our family. My mom taught us to never quit no matter how difficult the road ahead may seem.

BRADLEY (age 18), JACKIE'S SON

Two years ago, my Mom was diagnosed with breast cancer. The week before, I could tell something was wrong. I would see my mom pacing back and forth and becoming very irritable. Little did I know, earlier in the week she had felt a lump in her breast.

Things started making sense after my mom had a mammogram. From that, she learned she had a tumor in her breast, which could possibly be cancerous. Next, a long time friend of our family, Dr. David Applebaum, performed a biopsy on the tumor. He had the results almost instantly. As I saw my mom pulling into the driveway with tears pouring down her face, I knew something was wrong. It was a phone call from my dad that explained everything. He told me that my mom had cancer, he said not to worry, and that we were going to do everything and anything possible to get rid of it and keep her healthy! So the journey began!

Throughout the upcoming weeks it was doctor appointment after doctor appointment after doctor appointment, and all of them were giving us different information. To be honest, at that point I began to care less about what a doctor had to say about it and just wanted to find a way to help my mom. All of the big words the doctors used eventually led to me sitting at my computer "Googleing" everything and basically coming up with my own diagnosis. It was frustrating and upsetting.

Finally, my mom and the doctors came up with a treatment plan. She was going to have a double mastectomy and chemotherapy treatments. When I heard the word chemotherapy, the first thoughts in my mind were that my mom was going to loose her hair, screw up her memory and be in a lot of pain. I couldn't believe it. I kept thinking she shouldn't take the chemotherapy, it's not necessary. But, it was. At that point, I guess I was still in denial.

When the time came for my mom's chemotherapy to begin, I wanted to help her prepare for losing her hair. I worked in the mall at the time, so I knew of a store that sold wigs. Although, I didn't personally know anyone who needed a wig because they lost their hair, I did know of a lot of people that bought them as "fashion statements". At first I went with her to a few different wig places around town, but she couldn't find anything that looked like her. So, a little reluctantly, we went to the mall where I worked (and hung out). Once we were there, she began hysterically crying in the middle of the mall. I freaked out and walked away, embarrassed I guess. She ended up buying a wig at that store and thought it would be a great idea to walk around the mall with it on. It didn't quite work out that great, she was hysterically crying as she walked around the mall with the wig on. Things did get better though. Her hair stylist came over to our house and made the wig look exactly like her hair before; she even put a little clip in it like she had done in the past. I took a deep breath and hoped she was ready.

Then chemotherapy started. About two weeks into her treatments, her hair started to come out and she decided to shave the rest of it off. At the time, my mom was in a daze and often didn't seem to even realize what was going on. Throughout her chemotherapy treatments she tried different methods of dealing with the pain including sleeping pills, resting and exercise. In the beginning she wouldn't walk around the house without her wig on either. I know it was very upsetting to her to have lost her hair. Towards the end of her chemotherapy, though, she would pull into the garage and whip the wig off before she even got into the house.

Talking to my mom about cancer and her wearing a wig was the hardest part for me. I never knew what to say and what not to say. The unfortunate reality was there was nothing right to say. Nothing was going to make her feel better and nothing was going to help the pain; it was just a waiting game.

Once chemotherapy ended, I thought it would all be over, but it wasn't. Dealing with my mom waiting for her hair to grow back was a long process. It was hard for my mom to be patient and wait it out. She used every hair cream, oil or vitamin available to help her hair grow. Finally, when my mom's hair was about two inches long, she got hair extensions put on. Hair extensions are basically a wig strapped to your head. But to my mom it was her hair. As long as it was attached, it did the job. The extensions gave her a great confidence boost; it was like she was back to normal.

It's been a little over two years now since her battle with breast cancer started and I have moved to Colorado to attend the University of Colorado. Throughout the entire time I was living at home, I never cried about my mom's cancer. I felt I had to be strong, because if she saw me crying she would know I was worried!

My mom's cancer actually did have some benefits. I learned that life is not forever and to cherish it. Stay close with your family and friends, because you never know if something like this can happen. When I first moved out of my house I really started to feel the effects of the previous two years. At the beginning, I felt like I was useless, I felt like I couldn't support her when her hair was almost back, and most of all, it was difficult not being with her. But after a little bit of time I was able to understand and know that the cancer was gone. There was no point in worrying about it now. Still, to this day, it affects my everyday life.

STEVEN (age 20), JACKIE'S SON

When my mom was diagnosed with breast cancer, I was faced with the initial shock of realizing the mortality of my parents. However, with a mother so young, it blindsided me. She has always been the youngest mother of all my friends' parents, and she's also, before her diagnosis, one of the healthiest people I've known. Because of this, I saw her as this invincible super-human to whom I could relate as a friend in addition to all her motherly attributes. The first time a child has to deal with the mortality of his parents, it usually comes with old age and senility, and it all comes over time, so he's prepared. Instead of having 30 years of coping with this mortality, I had a few seconds. My girlfriend, being very close to the family, remembers feeling a sense of helplessness. She could not make me feel better about it, nor could she help my mom feel better about it, which was all she wanted to do.

But after the initial wave of emotions, I always had a positive feeling about the whole situation. I was really upset, and it was a great strain, but I always had the impression that it was going to be ok. I never felt that her life was in danger, even though it may have been, and I think that is due on a large part to our family dynamic. We are all so close-knit, and that was one of the pillars that I could lean on during the whole time.

Our family is unique in the fact that we are a unit. It was never that my mother was going through chemotherapy and that we were watching. It was that our family was going through it together. When you have four other people to lean on, it makes things a lot easier. The conversations were conducted with the word "we"; what are "we" going to do next? And I knew that she was going to get through it, and she handled it so well, so I wanted her to be proud of the cancer, or the fact that she overcame it. I wished that she had walked around without her wig on and faced it in public to teach everyone else that they could do it too and that she was so strong. It never even seemed like she was sick; she didn't throw up, and she only took her wig off in front of family. Incidentally, she happened to be the most beautiful bald woman in the world, and I wanted everyone to see her natural beauty. There's this negative stigma attached to cancer that its terrible and bleak, but I wanted people to understand that it can be uplifting to fight it. You can become stronger from the experience. I wanted people to realize that we were all determined, so everything was going to be fine, and we all knew it.

CINDY'S FRIEND RICHIE

For some reason, "cancer" is a word that I never really associated with youth. Growing up, I recall times when members of my family would be gathered around the table, speaking in hushed tones about how my grandmother or great aunt was "ill", as if somehow by whispering they could avoid awakening the disease. Cancer was discussed in conspiratorial tones, as if its victim had committed some egregious act that led in part to their illness or so it seemed to a child.

It's no wonder then, that I, and so many others of my generation, attributed "boogie-man" qualities to the disease. It was only in my mid-20, when my favorite aunt was diagnosed with breast cancer that I began to understand the disease more from an adult perspective. I watched as she battled her illness for 5 years and saw how it impacted her health, her spirit, and ultimately, her life.

Still, nothing can adequately prepare you for the day when someone close to you tells you those terrifying words "I have cancer". Every negative image, every fear real or imagined, all pass through your mind in the blink of an eye. When I learned that the person I was closest to in the world, Cindy, had cancer, I was stunned. Had she told me that she was giving birth to an alien I would have been no less affected. It just didn't register with anything I had convinced myself I knew about the disease. She wasn't old. She wasn't infirmed. She didn't have any contributory habits that would have placed her at high risk. She was (and is) the essence of youth, light, and vitality. The shock was especially hard because although a lump had been discovered, she had been "assured" that it was probably nothing and almost certainly benign. As she told me the news through tears on a cell-phone, I felt as if the earth beneath me had lost its permanence.

Those 48 hours were, without question, the hardest period of my life. I was confused. I was paralyzed with fear, both for my friend and for myself. I ran through the litany of inexorable questions, all the hows and whys, all in a vain and inevitably futile attempt to make sense of what had happened.

After the initial shock and concern, I realized that I had literally no idea what I was supposed to do. As it turned out, Cindy was the one (as always) to make it all clear. Within a week, she had acquired all of the information necessary to become a practicing oncologist. She knew the terminology, the various options for treatment, the timeline of events, and all of the probabilities and associated risks. She made information her ally and used it to reduce not only her own fear, but mine as well. Not only did she use the word "cancer" (gasp!) in conversation, she told me what role I was expected to play as part of her "love network".

And I realized that the more we all did, the more we all knew, and the more we all shared, the less fear I started to have. Not to say that I wasn't terrified—we all were—but by shining a light on the "boogey-man", by learning about it and talking about it, we were leveling the playing field, if only a bit.

What struck me the most at the time was the way in which Cindy led this charge and responded to her cancer. She didn't cower and retreat. She didn't let others manage this crisis for her. She didn't allow us to speak in the hushed tones I recalled from my youth. I am reminded of the Horace quote "Adversity reveals character" and nothing could have been truer.

Cindy's cancer was not hers alone. It impacted the lives of everyone around her—co-workers, friends, and family. We all experienced the fear and uncertainty, the sadness and tears, the frustration and anger, and eventually the sense of relief and hope that Cindy felt.

Cindy has advised me that she remains at a higher risk than most for a possible recurrence because she is BRCA 1 positive, so cancer is never truly defeated. At times, random events or some particular trigger will bring all of the fear and uncertainty to the forefront. But she doesn't let this fear control her. She doesn't put her life on hold. She knows who her friends are and she knows how much she is loved. She still supports her "sisters" who are going through the experiences with cancer that she went though. Cindy speaks more plainly these days—not afraid to express her love, not willing to put off the traveling she enjoys, not prepared to take a back seat and let life's journey pass her by. Cancer affected her body and health, but it never could change who she was. In this respect, she triumphed. When her head was bare, she was still the beautiful woman I had fallen in love with. She was still radiant. She still lit up a room just by walking in, and she still touched our hearts with her words and actions.

And I've learned things as well. Cindy's experience has taught me how strong one person can be, how it is possible to face even the greatest challenges and adversity, how fragile and precarious life can be. I know now that cancer is not a boogie-man; it's just a terrible disease that affects the lives of so many. I've learned that information and action serve as a better mentor than silence. I've learned that having a loving and supportive environment is key to maintaining your spirit and that telling and showing the people you love how much they mean to you serves as its own reward.

LISA, CINDY'S FRIEND

It started as an ordinary phone conversation between best friends. Catching up on the week's events, catching up on the ups and downs we faced that day, sharing funny stories and laughing the minutes away. Little did we know that ordinary night would be the beginning of my best friend's extraordinary year. As she laughed about sitting on her couch giving herself a breast exam, I laughed back and asked her if she found anything interesting. When she responded that she felt a rather large lump in one breast, our light conversation quickly changed to figuring out a serious plan of action that would start the very next day with a trip to the doctor. I am so grateful that on that ordinary day, Cindy unknowingly did a breast exam and took the first of many steps that would ultimately save her life.

From Chicago, I anxiously waited to hear what the "experts" thought about that crazy, large lump. I remember that feeling of relief when she told me all the "experts" felt it was nothing more than a large cyst, including the surgeon who removed it. I also remember sitting at the bank on a cold, rainy February afternoon when she called to tell me the "experts" were wrong … it was cancer and it was aggressive. I never made it into the bank.

Though I knew she would have a tough, grueling year ahead, I was so impressed at the way she kept making sure she looked out for her own well being right from the start. There are many women who would have stopped digging when they were told it was nothing to worry about, but not Cindy. She is a role model for young women, as well as a model of strength and courage for everyone.

Cindy's true colors and spirit were so prominent as she worked on her treatment plan, met other women who could mentor her, as well as becoming a mentor for other women who were behind her in their treatment plan. She always kept her sense of humor even when I know she was really terrified. She allowed her friends and family to support and love her, and I am so proud to have been one of the women she made part of her circle. She gathered us together a few days before her double mastectomy for a "boob" voyage celebration to celebrate the beginning of her cancer free life. She called us together to give her our strength and courage before the surgery. In truth, she gave us strength and courage just by being the amazing woman we all love.

How has fighting breast cancer changed my best friend? I think the process showed her how strong and capable she is as a woman. I think it helped her realize how much her family and friends love her. It gave her a way to support and share herself with other women who would not have otherwise come into her life. I hope that as the years go on, and she remains cancer free, she is able to conquer all her dreams with the same spirit and gusto that she demonstrated this past year as she fought the cancer.

Cindy and I are more than best friends. We are sisters. Thanks to her, we will be a part of each other's lives until we are old, gray-haired women swinging on a porch swing at a nursing home, and for that I am grateful. And of course, thanks to her amazing breast reconstruction, her boobs will still be perky and fabulous. I love you, Cindy.

SHARLA, TAMARA'S MOM

I am a mother of not one, but two daughters diagnosed with breast cancer. The "big C word", as my generation would say. I grew up associating cancer with a long struggle with illness and most often resulting in an untimely death.

When Tamara called her dad and me to tell us that she, too, had breast cancer (her sister had been diagnosed one month prior), I was in shock! I couldn't believe it. A million thoughts began running through my head. Why her? Why them? And, what did I do to cause this? We had never lived near any power lines, in fact most of the girls lives were spent with a lot of fresh air and "the great outdoors". They were raised as vegetarians and were always very active and healthy. We did not have a family history of breast cancer, so we assumed that they must have the genetic mutation for them both to get the disease.

When the results from the genetic testing came back negative for the BRCA1 and BRCA2 (identified breast cancer genes), we were speechless yet again.

However, regardless of how or why they ended up with breast cancer, they were still our "little girls": young, strong and with so much life left to live. After the initial shock, we dug in both feet and helped our daughters fight their cancers any way we could. We helped them determine the best plan of action was for each of them. We encouraged them to look not only at the short term, but the long term prognosis associated with each treatment plan. As much as possible, we tried to help ease their burdens of family life. Tamara's sister had a toddler to care for, and Tamara had been married only three short months. We tried to be supportive not only to the girls, but to their families too. We feel so fortunate that both girls had such strong support systems at home and that they had each other. We can already tell how this had impacted their relationship with each other and are grateful for the strong bond that they share.

It has been a very difficult journey for our daughters—journeys we wish we could have endured for them instead of with them. But our daughters have triumphed with flying colors. We are so proud of them. They are both so brave and strong. We are thankful to God for giving them a second chance at life and families still intact to share it with them.

SHAUNA, TAMARA'S SISTER

I am a corporate attorney living in Austin, Texas with my two year old son and husband. I was diagnosed with Stage II breast cancer on August 4, 2005 at the age of 33. I immediately had two surgeries related to removing my cancer tumor and the cancer from my lymph nodes. In addition, I had two surgeries to harvest eggs and freeze embryos for purposes of having more children. I completed nine months of chemotherapy last May 2006. As the final step in my treatment plan, I completed a bi-lateral mastectomy with immediate reconstruction in August 2006. My final reconstruction surgery took place in January 2007. Finally, after almost two years, my treatment for breast cancer is complete.

Two months into my treatment, Tamara called and said that she had breast cancer too. She was only 31 years old at the time. When I was diagnosed with breast cancer the first thing I did was call my sister and tell her that she should go get a mammogram. She did so immediately, and low and behold she too had the same invasive, ductal carcinoma cancer in her left breast that I had. Hers was at an earlier stage in that it had not spread into her lymph nodes as mine had. Although I realize that my diagnosis led to an earlier diagnosis of my sister's breast cancer and probably saved her life, I still felt somehow guilty and responsible for the pain that lay ahead for her. Over the last two years she has completed a similar course of treatment to mine, which also included bi-lateral mastectomy, reconstruction and chemotherapy.

My sister and I both lost all of our hair and our breasts. Talk about a serious bonding experience. My sister and I have always been close, but we now had new club of two. We built a support network of each other. We began to consult each other almost daily on everything from our treatments to what type and color of wig to buy, to the optimal time to shave your head to avoid the trauma of loosing it strand by strand. We would send each other flowers and cards. We were strong for each other and always a shoulder to cry on when things looked so dark. Breast cancer has changed our lives forever. Never again will we take each other for granted. We now make sure to call each other on a regular basis to talk about what is going on with our lives and take time out of our schedules to visit each other and spend quality time together.

PAUL, GINA'S HUSBAND

I remember that day like it was yesterday. The night before I had a sword fishing trip with some friends off Miami Beach, we were 25 miles offshore at 2 am and the Captain said, "If you hook one now, we're going to be out here all night." I said, "We better not, my wife has an important doctors appointment tomorrow, I need to be around." Turns out, I was right.

You never expect that phone call, and I cry every time I think about that moment, but hearing the woman I love telling me she had breast cancer was the single worst moment of my life. I'm not sure how we got through it. One day we're making vacation plans, and the next minute we're meeting surgeons. One minute, we're pinching ourselves because of the charmed lives we lead and the next minute my wife is losing her hair. It was a two year nightmare that never seemed to end.

At work, I always seemed to be able to handle any situation. If I lost a job, I'd easily find another one. I have always been in control of every situation that I found myself in, except this one. I was lost. Was I going to lose the light of my life? That wasn't in our plans. We were going to retire and cruise a boat up to Maine. Why did this happen? How was she going to survive it? How were the kids going to deal with it? How was I going to handle it?

When I first met Gina, I kept all my receipts in a huge cooler in the garage, had a pile of laundry that a small family could live in, and my refrigerator usually consisted of a half a gallon of milk and something unidentifiable in tin foil. She organized my life; she took care of me and helped me balance everything out. All of a sudden, she gets sick, we *still* have two kids and I *still* have a career, there was no way I was going to hold it all together. Thank God for friends and family.

If this ever happens to you or your family, everybody you know is going to say, "If there is anything I can do, just call". Don't be afraid to take them up on that. You've heard the expression, "That's what friends are for". Boy, are they ever. We had it down to a science, I left for work at 4:30 am, somebody was there to help get the kids off to school and take care of whatever Gina's needs were (most of the time it was one of the Grandma's). I would take over when I got home; pick up kids and then, the only good thing to come out of all this: The food would arrive!

Monday was Jill's night, Tuesday was Nancy's, Wednesday was somebody else, you get the picture. At about six o'clock every night, the door bell would ring and one of our closest friends would deliver enough food for an army. The kids would eat two chicken nuggets and some Mac n' cheese, Gina would attempt to nibble on whatever she could get down, and I would scarf up everything else.

Other friends who weren't on "the meal plan" didn't know what to do, so they would send over catered food. Anthony's Runway 84 and Café Maxx, two of the famous restaurants in South Florida, knew what was going on and were sending food over on a regular basis too. At one point, I didn't have enough room in the fridge. What a horrible problem to have! Once my wife was better, I asked her if we could just keep that wonderful news among ourselves, just so I could keep feeding. We didn't.

I've been a radio and TV personality in the Miami/Ft. Lauderdale area since 1984, and basically have lived my entire life on the radio. I do the morning show on Big 105.9, "The Paul and Young Ron show". People have known and continue to know everything (within reason) about my life. When I first met Gina was a big part of the show, when we got married, when our son was born, all of these things have become a part of "who I am" on the air. When we got Gina's news, we really didn't know what to do. First of all, I was a wreck. Try to do a comedy show when you feel that your life is falling apart around you; it ain't easy.

I'm a workaholic, and except for vacations, never take a day off from work. Thankfully, the company was terrific and said, "Do what you have to do for your family". I made sure I was with Gina during every one of the 800 doctor appointments she had during the first month or so. But it was obvious something was wrong. I wasn't myself, the show was suffering, I was missing work a lot, and after all those years on the air, the audience knew something wasn't right. Then Gina pulled me aside and made a huge decision that changed our lives and perhaps thousands of others. She decided to go public with her news.

The following morning at 8:30, and I will remember this moment in my career forever, I said I have a major announcement to make when I come back. I had already told my crew that I was going to be leaving at 9, but they had no idea what was coming next. I laid it on the line: through the tears I said, in a nutshell,

"Gina has breast cancer, and we're going to beat this thing". And I left to be with my wife.

I called her, we cried together, then I turned on the radio to listen to my partner Ron Brewer field call after call from concerned listeners and well wishers. How did that change our lives and the lives of others? I wouldn't realize that until days later when I began reading the literally thousands of e-mails that came pouring in.

Most of them were from people that have listened to my show for years and wanted to extend prayers and hope, but quite a few came from people that said, "My God, if it can happen to Paul and Gina, it can happen to anybody. I am going to make sure my wife, my sister and My Mom all go get checked out." Sadly, a few of those people came back later saying that they in fact did have breast cancer, but because of Gina's courage going public, it may have saved their loved one's life. That's pretty cool.

Earlier I asked, "How were we going to deal with it?" So far, we're three for three. Gina is the strongest, most awe inspiring person I have ever met. Sure we had a few bumps in the road during her treatment and recovery (one time I bought her the wrong type of burrito and she nearly killed me!), but guess what: she did it. My kids? Our youngest was 5 when she was diagnosed; and it seems Gina missed most of his kindergarten year. But you know what ... he barely has any recollection of her losing her hair, let alone being sick. Hopefully one day he won't have to think about it at all.

Our oldest son was in junior high, as tough as that is, add a sick Mom into the equation and that can spell trouble. I'm proud to say he made the honor roll in his first year of high school. Me, I gained a few pounds; got a few more gray hairs, but I have two things going for me: my wife is still here, I'm working on the extra pounds, and the two of us are getting ready to pick out that boat.

DOMANE, DONNA'S MOM

First of all, it is such a shock and heartbreak to learn that your daughter has cancer. You think that she is too young to go through this kind of trauma. I'm glad that I could be with her during this life altering experience in her life. A woman certainly needs a lot of support at a time like this, both in the hospital and at home. Just having someone close by to help you eat, get things out of reach, drain blood from the tubes, help you dress, driving to the doctor's office, etc. Donna was a trooper throughout this whole ordeal. Endless family support and prayers are equally important. I tried to provide the moral support, love and affection that only a mother can!

PATRICK, DONNA'S FRIEND

At a standing room only homeowner's association meeting in October of 2005 necessitated by the destruction caused by Wilma, I was fortunate enough to squeeze in next to an attractive and friendly woman by the name of Donna Palmisciano. Following the meeting, we exchanged small talk and business cards and that was the beginning of our friendship. Recently divorced, Donna was gearing up for, and adjusting to, her new "single" life. I was more that happy to spend time with her and we quickly became "fast friends". A feisty, petite and independent Italian girl, Donna is a compassionate, loyal, trustworthy and down to earth person who will always go out her way to help those in need. Everyone needs a "Donna" in their life!

We enjoyed the holidays together in 2005 and continued spending time together into the summer of 2006. In August, the news of Donna's diagnosis tore into our lives just like the hurricanes had the previous summer but this time with no warning! The first thought that crossed my mind was *"not again"*! I had just been through a similar scenario in December 2004 with another very close friend. But just like any other disaster, it's all about the recovery effort, so, it was time to roll up our sleeves and get to work.

The good news, if there is any such a thing as good news in a situation like this, is that I was very familiar with the deluge that was about to overtake Donna's life. Hopefully, this experience was helpful in instilling a sense of calmness and comfort for Donna as she prepared for upcoming barrage of tests, appointments and treatments that would be coming her way in the weeks and months ahead. I tried to be the buffer and sounding board for the myriad of decisions that were made regarding all the treatment protocols. I hoped that my prior experience could be used to make Donna feel a little safer in her decision making process. I tried to constantly reassure her that she was making the right decisions.

True to form, Donna remained extremely independent and strong throughout the entire treatment process. I still to this day marvel at her courage, strength and sheer determination. From time to time, I found myself tentative and not sure how best to "participate" in her treatment and recovery phases. There is a fine line between honoring one's desire to be independent and acting on my instinct to help in any way possible. Sometimes, I did not feel that I was "present enough" during certain phases of her treatments. Today, I would handle things a little differently if faced with a similar situation. Strong and independent is great but so is the feeling of safety and security derived from the constant presence of your "rock". Phone calls to check up are comforting but nothing can replace a warm caress or a gentle hug to help make you feel better. The human element is extremely important in the healing process and I do not think that I was there enough for Donna in this regard.

I also sensed a desire from both the "patient" and the "caregiver" perspective to maintain a normalcy in our everyday lives. Balance is the key! Donna tenaciously maintained a full professional schedule while enduring the physical demands of the treatment protocols. I am not sure if there is a "correct" answer to the dilemma of working and healing, however, I strongly encourage any patient wanting to maintain their independence to allow friends into your space to help as much as possible. There will be plenty of time in the future to be on your own, so take advantage of your support systems as much as possible.

Another significant element in the healing process is the mental and emotional aspect that can be easily overlooked. Long after the bandages are gone, the port removed and the wig has been pitched into the Halloween costume box, the need for continued support remains. Make time to listen. I strongly encourage all caregivers to remain steadfast in your commitment to your loved ones and realize that a sympathetic ear or a simple "how a you feeling today?" can serve as an important conduit to the continued healing for our loved ones. And after all treatments are over, always remember that the three most under prescribed drugs are faith, hope and love! Give all that you can; their addiction is painless and the side effects are wonderful.

As you can see, a breast cancer diagnosis impacts the entire family, and more often than not, the whole community. It is very real and present in our lives. Our sisterhood is growing as we speak. It is vital that we continue to share our stories and support one another. It is also important to raise awareness and educate. Then, and only then, is the possibility for a cure in our future.

CHAPTER SEVEN

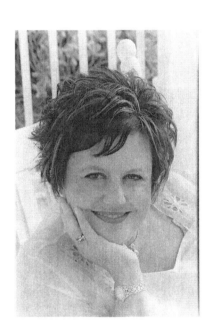
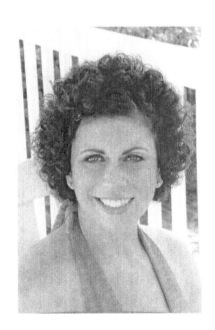

LIFE AFTER

"I had heard that the end of chemotherapy is kind of a let down. I wasn't sure what people meant. Now I know. Chemotherapy is like a marathon. You pace yourself and gain comfort in the routine. Knowing what doctors you'll see and what you'll feel like. Once the race is over, there is a moment of "OK, what now?" What had become familiar evolves into the unfamiliar land of waiting. Waiting to get my period back, waiting for my hair to grow, waiting to finish reconstruction, waiting for follow up appointments ..."

—Cindy

Moving on once your treatments are over is yet one other major adjustment that must be made. Fitting back into a lifestyle that you were so abruptly removed from is challenging at best. Our transition from being a cancer patient to that of a survivor and once again, wife, mother, daughter, sister or friend began with baby steps. Allow yourself a chance to breathe and to reflect on the journey you have just traveled. You are moving back in the driver's seat and a healthy, long, good life is in the destination. You have been given the tools, strength and courage through your experience to achieve your dreams and desires. The rest is truly up to you.

THE TRANSITION

"For months I was constantly going from one doctor appointment to another. It was exhausting. I felt like I had a full time job as an architect and a part-time job as a cancer patient."

—*Donna*

DONNA

I felt I was no longer a "patient" when all my treatments stopped. You are going and going for months from one doctor's appointment to the next and it can be exhausting. I have a full time job as an architect and a part-time job as a cancer patient. It sometimes felt like a dream that I was acting in. I remember the time I was sitting in a doctor's waiting room, I would think to myself, "I can't believe I had cancer! I am a young, healthy and vibrant person; I don't belong here among the sick." As I would look around the waiting room, I realized that I had it so much better than some of the other people in the room. I never forget that it could be so much worse. Through all of this, I never got mad at God. I am grateful that I have been very healthy up to this point in my life. God doesn't promise us a perfect life without struggles. I guess it was my turn. My body was put to the test, my character was strengthened and all my senses where heightened. I'm almost grateful that it was breast cancer vs. some other type of cancer. When caught early enough, breast cancer is one of the better cancers to have with a good survival rate.

My transition back to "normal" life was nothing close to normal. Many cancer survivors refer to life after cancer as the "new normal". After going through the experience of breast cancer, you are forever changed! You will never be totally the same 'ol you again. I like to think that I'm a better person because of the experience.

Physically, I used to exercise at the gym regularly before the cancer came into my life. I am finding it hard to get back to the gym on a regular basis. I still have some joint pain, so when I'm stretching and lifting weights I feel the pain. They say "no pain, no gain". I'm trying to work through the pain but I find I want to quit when it hurts. I am trying to build up my endurance and strength again. It's amazing how much strength I lost. I had a hard time just opening up a jar! But, I am determined to get back into shape again. Exercising and keeping yourself at a good weight is crucial for cancer patients. I feel that it will help my self-esteem and my body image if I can get into great shape. On top of all that, my reconstruction is not complete yet. I'm still waiting for my nipples and hope I get them for Christmas!

Being a single person again after a long marriage, I find that it's hard to date. I want to date and be in a caring relationship but I have to deal with a lot of new issues that I didn't have before. One issue that I have to deal with now is, when is the "right time" to tell someone about my cancer? Too soon and it may scare them off, too late and they may feel like I was hiding something and not being honest up front. Some guys may be scared and think that the cancer may come back and don't want to get involved with me. I believe that I will find a great guy that will love and accept me with all my flaws both physically and emotionally.

Emotionally, I try to stay positive and believe that my cancer will not come back. But, in the back of my mind that thought surfaces once in a while. It makes me think twice now when making some decisions. In the months following the completion of my treatments, I experienced the "FUNK". I was feeling depressed and couldn't shake it. I still can't pinpoint the exact cause of my depression. It may be a side effect of Tamoxifen, or my lack of exercise, raging hormones, or the feeling you get when the whirlwind comes to a complete stop. Maybe subconsciously I was upset about having had cancer. I may never know exactly what it was. It was probably a combination of all the above. The good news is that I'm finally starting to feel better, getting back to the gym, coming out of the funk and looking forward to an exciting future. There are still many things that I want to do and experience in my remaining time on this earth. Godspeed.

DEBBIE

For me, life after began with my adjustment to having short hair. I had to find a new and attractive short hair cut and style, in order to recover my self confidence. It didn't happen all at once but eventually I found the right hairdresser and the right style for me. Then, I had the challenge of putting things into perspective and started working on maintaining a healthy lifestyle.

Within minutes of being diagnosed with breast cancer, I felt as if I was thrust onto a roller coaster already in motion. My "ride" stopped only for surgeries, treatments, blood tests and doctor appointments. The highs and lows all blurred together and life during that time passed me by. Then, as abruptly as the ride had begun, it was over.

I was left with my life, a wonderful husband and family, a pill (Tamoxifen), a wig (there would be no hair for months), and what seemed like forever until my next doctor appointment.

I was now expected to resume my life where I had left off as if the past year was just a bad dream. Only it wasn't a dream. It was real, and it was impossible for everything to continue exactly as it was before. I had new challenges to face, and I had to continue to take care of myself and my family in new ways.

"I have finished all of my treatments" was something I heard myself saying often, but inside I was thinking, "Now what?" "What do I do?" "How do I move forward?" I have no hair. I still don't feel right. It felt as if everyone was acting like there had been a broken switch that got repaired and didn't understand how I wasn't able to "get with the program". Weren't I happy to be alive and a part of life?

The answer, of course, is "yes". I was happy to be finished with my treatments and my surgeries and to not be rushing from one doctor appointment to another.

So, I began with baby steps. I slowly resumed my life. I started with my husband and children, parents and friends: actively participating in their lives, encouraging, nurturing and caring for them with a whole new perspective on life and how I wanted to live it. As I became more comfortable and confident about rejoining society, I took off my wig approximately four months after my last chemotherapy treatment. It took a lot of courage. I had lived 37 years with long hair and now I was going to walk out the door with hair that was about three inches long. Looking back, I am so thankful that I was able to do it. Largely, the support of my husband and children (who are always honest about appearance) gave me the confidence to do it. As silly as it sounds, I have learned many incredible lessons about myself, the people around me and how others perceive me by "owning my short hair".

I have also become much better at putting things into perspective. I feel I am better at sorting out what is important and what's not—lessons I hope to instill in my children. I hope to teach them to be less judgmental, more caring of themselves and others and to appreciate the gift of life.

Lastly, I realize the need to lead a healthy lifestyle for myself and my family. This has come about, not from having cancer, but from my parents. Their determination to find a way to "help" has profoundly affected our family. Due to their insistency and consistency in teaching us, even my young children, about eating to live, not living to eat we are all feeling better. I see it with my husband. I notice it in my children, and I feel it for myself.

It's not easy in a world where convenience is key and time is at a premium. Even exercise has to fit into the schedule. However, eating healthy and exercise has become part of our vocabulary and conversation in my home. My children are asking for carrots instead of cookies and the lowering of my husband's blood pressure are signals that a healthy diet and lifestyle work. It's all part of the package to live a long life, feel good physically and mentally and allow yourself to love and be loved.

TAMARA

Sometimes, I look back and I wonder what took more strength to get through. Did the surgery and chemotherapy seem as hard to get through as the period when it was over? I remember being in fight mode during my treatments. It was all about taking the next step. Get through it and just survive. It became automatic. I don't think that I dealt with it emotionally during that time. I was in denial, as weird as that sounds.

It finally hit me when I finished the core doses of my chemotherapy. It is at this time, that everyone around you, even your spouse, breathes a collective sigh of relief and says, "It's over. You are fine now." From a cancer patient's perspective, this is the most ridiculous statement ever made. Of course I am not fine now. I still have all the residual problems left over from chemotherapy. I am emotionally unstable, for a number of reasons. My menstrual cycle has come back causing a huge, unpredictable hormonal imbalance that I could not control with birth control pills as I used to. I was depressed each time I had to return to the CTU (chemotherapy treatment unit) to receive my Herceptin infusion, and my daily dose of Tamoxifen wasn't a happy reminder either. These two drugs were "a hard pill to swallow", as they say, not to mention the side effects. Although I was happy to have hair again, we all know how painful the growing out process can be. I was working triple time in the gym to try to get my body back. On top of all that it finally hit me, "I had cancer!"

I went through a very rough emotional patch, which I can only describe as post-traumatic stress syndrome. At one point I thought I would end up divorced and in a mental institution. I had to get help! I went to see the counselor that is provided by the hospital and also runs our support group. She helped me to sort out a lot of my emotions and get through the worst of it. Many of my doctors' recommended taking an antidepressant. For a long time, I refused to take any more medications. I was worried about more side effects and I also wanted to face and deal with cancer and not cover it up with "happy pills".

When I completed my year of Herceptin treatments, I felt a dramatic improvement in my overall mood. Still, many things bothered me. Finally, after several months I gave in and allowed myself to take an antidepressant. I was prescribed Lexapro which is an antidepressant that is often used to treat women with menopausal and hormonal side effects. I am happy to say that it has helped a great deal and I am feeling much more normal again.

It is very difficult to be faced with everyone telling you and acting like you are normal again. In truth we have just begun our lifelong journey with breast cancer. There needs to be a time of adjustment. As someone once said, "I had cancer, it does not have me!"

GINA

People say you are a survivor from the moment you are told you have cancer. Some survivors even refer to their diagnosis day as their birthday. Although I love my birthday as never before, I'm going to stick to one a year. For me, "life after" is an attempt to move forward with some normalcy while using my experiences to effect change in my life and the lives of others. I have also embraced a quiet activism in a way that suits my life style.

As previously mentioned, I am married to Paul who hosts a radio show in South Florida. He also works in television and writes a magazine column. Because of our visibility and willingness to share our experience, the announcement of my illness drove home the need for early detection. We know of women who were moved to get checked and were subsequently diagnosed. Paul has also used his show to raise money for cancer research. At public appearances I've tried to put on a brave face so others can see that survivors are whole people; even though it involves an occasional uncomfortable stare or awkward moment.

When the local ABC television affiliate asked us if they could tell our story, we willingly let them into our lives. We took the spotlight, which is normally focused on him, and redirected it to shine on something important. I even let the cameras follow me to my first radiation treatment. Together we helped to raise awareness about breast cancer. We attempted to reach the women who don't get mammograms because they are too afraid of the outcome. Our message was: It can happen to anyone, and when it does, you move forward with the love and support of your family. You can survive.

Politically, I feel a sense of responsibility to speak out on behalf of all the women who have been and will be affected by this disease. Currently, this number is one in eight. I will always be grateful to those that have come before me—the women who raised money for research, the women who volunteered to participate in drug trials and the women who fought for better care from insurance companies. In honor of them, I recently spoke up. It took a little effort and a lot of determination, but I am so proud I did it! I had the opportunity to meet Nancy Pelosi, Speaker of the House of Representatives and third in line to the presidency. There was one problem however; I was scheduled for reconstruction surgery just two days before the political event. It was to be my sixth and final surgery and to reschedule would mean I would have to endure another summer without my nipples. Normally the dressing used by the surgeon would prevent the patient from wearing a cocktail dress for about a week. This was unacceptable. I begged my plastic surgeon to think of another way to bandage me up, and he did. Forty-eight hours later, I was all dressed up and headed to the Diplomat Hotel. I had something to say.

As I stood in line waiting to meet Speaker Pelosi, everyone around me was busy getting their cameras ready for the photo op. I had no camera; there would be no time for that. Finally it was my turn. I said, "Nancy I don't want a picture with you, I just came here to tell you something." Her attention was mine, so I continued, "I'm a breast cancer survivor of 18 months, I had surgery 48 hours ago and my surgeon bandaged me up so I could come here to ask you to keep fighting for stem cell research." The Speaker's eyes widened. For a moment it seemed as if everyone around us disappeared. Her security guards and handlers were no longer in focus. Her facial expression quickly went from surprise to concern. She grabbed my hands, asked me my name and gave me a little hug. "God bless you and good luck," she said. Within minutes she was whisked away. I headed home as well, happy I hadn't let the opportunity to be heard pass me by.

Every day as a survivor I attempt to live joyfully and not let the fear of recurrence dominate my thoughts. I am incredibly grateful for my life. I don't want to put off living out my dreams, pursuing them with a new sense of urgency and passion. I try to take advantage of the opportunities that present themselves to me, even if it's an opportunity to play a board game with my son. My family and I recently went to Italy. We also went to the Super Bowl, something I have wanted to do for the longest time. As Billy Joel belted out the National Anthem from the center of Dolphin Stadium, the tears welled up in my eyes. I glanced at my husband and his eyes were wet too. Without saying anything, he reached for my hand and gave it a squeeze. We had made it, and there were so many great things yet to come!

JACKIE

After my treatments ended, life has been a slow but uplifting journey. The further I get from my treatments, the more spread out my doctor appointments become, the longer my hair gets, the better I feel. I appreciate life more. I take time to enjoy many of the things I would have put off until another day prior to my breast cancer diagnosis.

I have always made time for my family; they are the core of my being. However, now, I feel like I am seeing them in a new light. I feel as if I am truly experiencing their lives with them. I feel even more connected to them than I ever thought possible. I cherish the simple things and welcome the challenges of life.

I make it a point not to dwell on my cancer treatments. I want to continue to move forward and not waste another moment. When I first got diagnosed I knew I wasn't ready to throw in the towel. I have been given a second chance at life and I'm not going to waste it!

CINDY

I had heard that the end of chemotherapy is kind of a let down. I wasn't sure what people meant. Now I know. Chemotherapy is like a marathon. You pace yourself and gain comfort in the routine—knowing what doctors you'll see and what you'll feel like. Once the race is over, there is a moment of—"OK, what now?" What had become familiar segues into the unfamiliar land of "Waiting." I was waiting to get my period back, waiting for my hair to grow, waiting to finish reconstruction, waiting for follow up appointments every three months. Waiting to deal with the BRCA 1 issues like a higher risk for ovarian cancer.

July 2007 marked the one year anniversary of the end of my chemotherapy. During that year I experienced a range of emotions—relief, fear of recurrence, mild depression, post traumatic stress, reevaluating my life, my purpose, my goals and much joy.

I know I'm different from this experience. My body is different, my hair is different, my sense of awareness is different. (Was there always so much cancer in the news, on television, in magazines?) It took about four months for my period to return and my hot flashes to subside. My hair is still a work in progress. The only part of my breast reconstruction left is the second and final areola tattooing.

Being one of the "single" girls in this club can be challenging. I think about all things my significant other may have to hear about and deal with to be in a relationship with me.

Because of my BRCA 1 status, I undergo trans-vaginal ultrasounds every three months. I know that I am on a deadline to decide if I want to have children. I need to remove my ovaries before I turn 44 to help reduce my very real risk of ovarian cancer. I still visit my Oncologist every three months for blood work and checkups.

People ask if I feel different and I do—sometimes. Sometimes, I slow down and see the world a little crisper, a little brighter. I sense people's energy now.

Sometimes my patience runs much shorter than it used to and sometimes I am humbled by the kindness of humanity.

There are days that my cancer is prevalent in my thoughts, and days that it is a mere thought as I see my breasts, my scars, my curly hair and realize that I am good, I look good and my life is good.

SEX

"Sex became a challenge for my husband and me. A new learning curve was in place. Slowly with practice, we found our way back to intimacy."

—*Gina*

GINA

My husband and I were married for nine years before my cancer diagnosis. With two children and a busy social schedule, we had what I considered a normal sex life. Then came the year of the drought. Although I did not have my mastectomy for five moths after my diagnosis, I was feeling pretty sick from the chemotherapy treatments. My hormones were raging, and I was an emotional wreck. When I did summon up the drive or guilt to have sex with my husband, my breasts quickly became off limits. The moment he touched me there, my mind went right to my illness. No matter what my body was saying, my mind would remember the tumor—still there, still a threat. No longer friends, my breasts gave new meaning to sleeping with the enemy. Sex became a challenge for my husband and me. A new learning curve was in place. Slowly with practice and a lot of lube, we found our way back to intimacy. I learned to let go and he learned to be patient. Even now, I find I prefer to keep my breasts out of play, covered with a teddy or sexy bra. In time, perhaps they'll find their way back into our repertoire.

Recently, I was counseling a newly diagnosed woman. She told me how worried she was to have a mastectomy, afraid that her sex life would be affected by the chest numbing surgery. I remember telling her, "You can't have sex if you are dead." I meant it. Our first priority is to live, all the other stuff will work itself out.

"Suddenly I went from being this happy, fun, sexy girl with a good body and long gorgeous hair, to a bald, cranky, and sick, out of shape, woman with funny looking boobs and a very painful dry vagina."

—*Tamara*

TAMARA

It becomes very difficult not only to physically have sex but mentally as well. We all know that for women, sex is very emotional and mental. If we don't feel good about ourselves, we are not interested. This is a particularly hard subject for me. My husband and I were newly married (three months) when I was diagnosed with breast cancer. Suddenly I went from being this happy, fun, sexy girl with a good body and long gorgeous hair, to a bald, cranky, and sick, out of shape, woman with funny looking boobs and a very painful dry vagina. There was no way I was having sex. It was very tough for both of us because I felt so guilty that he had married me and now I was the opposite of what he wanted. He couldn't even have sex with his wife for almost a year! I was very scared that he would want to leave me.

Fortunately, I married a wonderful man. He stuck by me. I tried to help him out as much as possible to at least give him some relief and help keep that intimacy between us that is only achieved by making love. Eventually, I was able to physically have sex and emotionally I am getting back to that place. I feel much better about myself and that helps. My advice is to make sure you keep up the intimacy. Both partners need it. Even if you don't have sex, enjoy each other in other ways. Remember, we may be going through hell, but so are our husbands.

CINDY

I was amazed that during this period I still had a sense of my self as a sexual being and even more amazed that I could still feel beautiful, sexy, and desirable. I'm sure that mostly had to do with the love and support of the man in my life.

To date, my sexual desire and drive continue to play an active role in my life. I am lucky to have never lost this part of myself.

As you find your way in life after breast cancer, be proud of what you have achieved. You are strong, brave, courageous and empowered. You have acquired gifts many go a lifetime and never receive. Give yourself credit for all you have accomplished and achieved. You earned it, and more importantly, you deserve it.

We hope that our book has informed, enlightened and uplifted the spirits of those affected by a breast cancer diagnosis. From the patient to the caregiver, we are all in this together. You are not alone.

As our mentor and friend, Darci McNally said, *"You are not an anomaly. It is not why me? Rather, why not you, or me or anyone? The good news is the technology for detection and treatment is has advanced greatly over the past decade and continues to do so as we speak. Get educated, get support and keep on living. You can't control the fact that you got cancer, but you can control how much it controls your life!!"*

978-0-595-45926-
0-595-45926-9

Printed in the United States
115549LV00004B/258/P

9 780595 459261